Developing an Empirically Based Practice Initiative: A Case Study in CPS Supervision

Developing an Empirically Based Practice Initiative: A Case Study in CPS Supervision has been co-published simultaneously as *Journal of Evidence-Based Social Work,* Volume 4, Numbers 3/4 2007.

Monographic Separates from the *Journal of Evidence-Based Social Work*™

For additional information on these and other Haworth Press titles, including descriptions, tables of contents, reviews, and prices, use the QuickSearch catalog at http://www.HaworthPress.com.

Developing an Empirically Based Practice Initiative: A Case Study in CPS Supervision, edited by Jenny L. Jones, PhD, and Paul Sundet, PhD (Vol. 4, No. 3/4, 2007). *Examines the integration of technology with evidence-based social work research, practice, and education.*

Building Excellence: The Rewards and Challenges of Integrating Research into the Undergraduate Curriculum, edited by Catherine N. Dulmus, PhD, and Karen M. Sowers, PhD (Vol. 4, No. 1/2, 2007). *A handbook for teaching undergraduate students to develop, use, and communicate research, using the curriculum of The University of Tennessee, College of Social Work as an example.*

Information Technology and Evidence-Based Social Work Practice, edited by Judith M. Dunlop, PhD, and Michael J. Holosko, PhD (Vol. 3, No. 3/4, 2006). *Examines the integration of technology with evidence-based social work research, practice, and education.*

Juvenile Offenders and Mental Illness: I Know Why the Caged Bird Cries, edited by Lisa A. Rapp-Paglicci, PhD, MSW (Vol. 2, No. 3/4, 2005). *A comprehensive compilation of experts' research and treatment strategies for juvenile offenders who have a mental illness.*

Addiction, Assessment, and Treatment with Adolescents, Adults, and Families, edited by Carolyn Hilarski, PhD (Vol. 2, No. 1/2, 2005). *An overview of current theory and practice concerning addiction treatment and assessment issues for all populations.*

Kids and Violence: The Invisible School Experience, edited by Catherine N. Dulmus, PhD, and Karen M. Sowers, PhD (Vol. 1, No. 2/3, 2004). *"Important.... will benefit school adminstrators, counselors, teachers, and personnel as they come to identify, understand, and act on violence in school settings." (Peter A. Newcombe, PhD, BEd, BA (Hons), Acting Program Director, Behavioural Studies, School of Social Work and Applied Human Sciences, The University of Queensland, Australia)*

Developing an Empirically Based Practice Initiative: A Case Study in CPS Supervision

Jenny L. Jones, PhD
Paul Sundet, PhD
Editors

Developing an Empirically Based Practice Initiative: A Case Study in CPS Supervision has been co-published simultaneously as *Journal of Evidence-Based Social Work,* Volume 4, Numbers 3/4 2007.

The Haworth Press, Inc.

www.HaworthPress.com

Developing an Empirically Based Practice Initiative: A Case Study in CPS Supervision has been co-published simultaneously as *Journal of Evidence-Based Social Work,* Volume 4, Numbers 3/4 2007.

Library of Congress Catalog-in-Publication Data

Developing an Empirically Based Practice Initiative: A Case Study in CPS Supervision/ Jenny L. Jones, PhD and Dr. Paul Sundet, editors.

p. cm.

"A Case Study in CPS Supervision has been co published simultaneously as Journal of Evidence-Based Social Work, Volume 4, Numbers 3/4 2007."

Includes bibliographical references and index.

ISBN 978-0-7890-3345-1 (hard cover : alk. paper) – ISBN 978-0-7890-3346-8 (soft cover : alk. paper)

1. Child welfare–Southern States–Management. 2. Child welfare–Management–Case studies. I. Jones, Jenny L. II. Sundet, Paul A. III. Journal of evdience-based social work.

HV742.S85D48 2008

362.70975–dc22 2007031311

The HAWORTH PRESS *Inc*

Abstracting, Indexing & Outward Linking

PRINT *and* ELECTRONIC BOOKS & JOURNALS

This section provides you with a list of major indexing & abstracting services and other tools for bibliographic access. That is to say, each service began covering this periodical during the year noted in the right column. Most Websites which are listed below have indicated that they will either post, disseminate, compile, archive, cite or alert their own Website users with research-based content from this work. (This list is as current as the copyright date of this publication.)

Abstracting, Website/Indexing Coverage	Year When Coverage Began
• *(IBR) International Bibliography of Book Reviews on the Humanities and Social Sciences (Thomson) <http://www.saur.de>*	**2006**
• ***Academic Search Premier (EBSCO)** <http://search.ebscohost.com>*	**2006**
• ***CINAHL (Cumulative Index to Nursing & Allied Health Literature) (EBSCO)** <http://www.cinahl.com>*	**2005**
• ***CINAHL Plus (EBSCO)** <http://search.ebscohost.com>*	**2006**
• ***MEDLINE (National Library of Medicine)** <http://www.nlm.nih.gov>*	**2007**
• ***Social Services Abstracts (ProQuest CSA)** <http://www.csa.com>*	**2004**
• ***Social Work Abstracts (NASW)** <http://www.silverplatter.com/catalog/swab.htm>*	**2006**
• *Academic Source Premier (EBSCO) <http://search.ebscohost.com>*	**2007**
• *Cambridge Scientific Abstracts (now ProQuest CSA) <http://www.csa.com>*	**2006**
• *Child Welfare Information Gateway (formerly National Adoption Information Clearinghouse Documents Database, and formerly National Adoption Information Clearinghouse on Child Abuse & Neglect Information Documents Database) <http://www.childwelfare.gov>*	**2006**
• *Criminal Justice Abstracts (Sage & CSA)*	**2006**

(continued)

- *Current Abstracts (EBSCO) <http://search.ebscohost.com>* **2007**
- *DH-Data (available via DataStar and in the HMIC [Health Management Information Consortium] CD ROM) <http://www.dh.gov.uk/Home/fs/en>* **2005**
- *EBSCOhost Electronic Journals Service (EJS) <http://search.ebscohost.com>* **2004**
- *Education Research Complete (EBSCO) <http://search.ebscohost.com>* **2006**
- *Education Research Index (EBSCO) <http://search.ebscohost.com>* . . **2007**
- *Electronic Collections Online (OCLC) <http://www.oclc.org/electroniccollections/>* **2006**
- *Elsevier Eflow -D <http://www.elsevier.com>* **2006**
- *Elsevier Scopus <http://www.info.scopus.com>* **2005**
- *Family & Society Studies Worldwide (NISC USA) <http://www.nisc.com>* **2003**
- *Family Index Database <http://www.familyscholar.com>* **2004**
- *Family Violence & Sexual Assault Bulletin>* **2006**
- *Google <http://www.google.com>* **2004**
- *Google Scholar <http://scholar.google.com>* **2004**
- *Haworth Document Delivery Center <http://www.HaworthPress.com/journals/dds.asp>* **2004**
- *IndexCopernicus <http://www.indexcopernicus.com>* **2007**
- *Information for Practice <http://www.nyu.edu/socialwork/ip/>* **2007**
- *International Bibliography of Periodical Literature on the Humanities and Social Sciences (IBZ) (Thomson) <http://www.saur.de>* **2006**
- *JournalSeek <http://www.journalseek.net>* **2006**
- *Links@Ovid (via CrossRef targeted DOI links) <http://www.ovid.com>* **2005**
- *NewJour (Electronic Journals & Newsletters) <http://gort.ucsd.edu/newjour/>* **2006**
- *OCLC ArticleFirst <http://www.oclc.org/services/databases/>* **2006**
- *Ovid Linksolver (OpenURL link resolver via CrossRef targeted DOI links) <http://www.linksolver.com>* **2005**
- *PSYCLINE <http://www.psycline.org>* **2006**
- *Sage Family Studies Abstracts* **2004**

(continued)

- *Scopus (See instead Elsevier Scopus) <http://www.info.scopus.com>* **2005**
- *Social Care Online (formerly CareData) <http://www.elsc.org.uk>* **2004**
- *Sociedad Iberoamericana de Información Científica (SIIC) <http://www.siicsalud.com/>* **2004**
- *SocIndex (EBSCO) <http://search.ebscohost.com>* **2006**
- *SocINDEX with Full Text (EBSCO) <http://search.ebscohost.com>* . . . **2007**
- *Special Educational Needs Abstracts>* **2006**
- *TOC Premier (EBSCO) <http://search.ebscohost.com>* **2007**
- *Women, Girls & Criminal Justice Newsletter (Civic Research Institute)>* **2004**

Bibliographic Access

- *MedBioWorld <http://www.medbioworld.com>*
- *MediaFinder <http://www.mediafinder.com/>*
- *Ulrich's Periodicals Directory: The Global Source for Periodicals Information Since 1932 <http://www.bowkerlink.com>*

Special Bibliographic Notes related to special journal issues (separates) and indexing/abstracting:

- indexing/abstracting services in this list will also cover material in any "separate" that is co-published simultaneously with Haworth's special thematic journal issue or DocuSerial. Indexing/abstracting usually covers material at the article/chapter level.
- monographic co-editions are intended for either non-subscribers or libraries which intend to purchase a second copy for their circulating collections.
- monographic co-editions are reported to all jobbers/wholesalers/approval plans. The source journal is listed as the "series" to assist the prevention of duplicate purchasing in the same manner utilized for books-in-series.
- to facilitate user/access services all indexing/abstracting services are encouraged to utilize the co-indexing entry note indicated at the bottom of the first page of each article/chapter/contribution.
- this is intended to assist a library user of any reference tool (whether print, electronic, online, or CD-ROM) to locate the monographic version if the library has purchased this version but not a subscription to the source journal.
- individual articles/chapters in any Haworth publication are also available through the Haworth Document Delivery Service (HDDS).

As part of Haworth's continuing commitment to better serve our library patrons, we are proud to be working with the following electronic services:

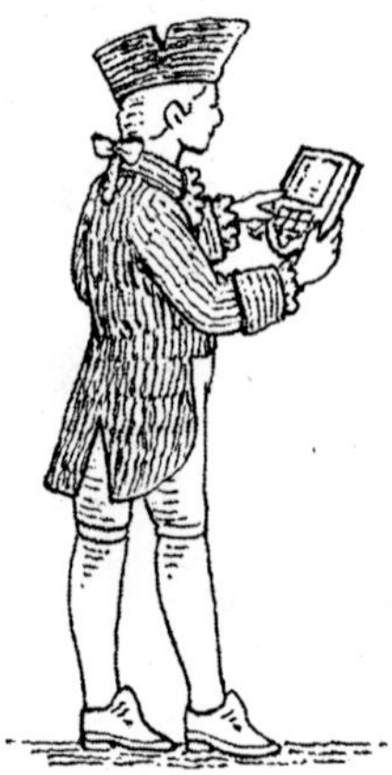

AGGREGATOR SERVICES

EBSCOhost

Ingenta

J-Gate

Minerva

OCLC FirstSearch

Oxmill

SwetsWise

LINK RESOLVER SERVICES

1Cate (Openly Informatics)

ChemPort (American Chemical Society)

CrossRef

Gold Rush (Coalliance)

LinkOut (PubMed)

LINKplus (Atypon)

LinkSolver (Ovid)

LinkSource with A-to-Z (EBSCO)

Resource Linker (Ulrich)

SerialsSolutions (ProQuest)

SFX (Ex Libris)

Sirsi Resolver (SirsiDynix)

Tour (TDnet)

Vlink (Extensity, formerly Geac)

WebBridge (Innovative Interfaces)

ABOUT THE EDITORS

Jenny L. Jones, PhD, is Assistant Professor in the College of Social Work at the University of Tennessee. She received her baccalaureate degree in psychology from Valdosta State (College) University in 1979, the Master Degree in Social Work from California State University Long Beach in 1990, and the PhD degree in Social Welfare from Clark Atlanta University in 2002. Dr. Jones' research focuses on child welfare policy, supervision, organizational culture, and intervention (to include mental health needs of AIDS-affected children and families). She has authored or co-authored several articles and book chapters, and has presented her research nationally and internationally. Prior to obtaining her PhD, her social work practice background encompassed over a decade of experience in the field of child welfare as a direct practitioner, administrator, and consultant.

Paul Sundet, PhD, is Professor Emeritus in the school of social work at the University of Missouri. He received his Master of Social Work degree from the University of Missouri and his doctorate from the School of Social Work, University of Illinois, Urbana-Champaign. His research and publications are in the areas of human service administration and management, rural human services and community mental health. His practice background includes child welfare, juvenile justice and mental health. In continuing education he has presented workshops to practitioners in twenty-seven states and three provinces. He is consultant to numerous state agencies and the legislature on issues of human service policy and program.

∞ ALL HAWORTH BOOKS AND JOURNALS
ARE PRINTED ON CERTIFIED
ACID-FREE PAPER

Developing an Empirically Based Practice Inititative: A Case Study in CPS Supervision

CONTENTS

Foreword

When the four state's child protective services supervisor demonstration training projects that serve as the context for the articles in this issue began, all recognized that researching the impact of the intervention models was both a requirement and a challenge. However, it is doubtful that any of the participants foresaw the complexity of implementing both an internal experimental/control design within their own jurisdiction and simultaneously complying with conditions of cross-site evaluation. In all instances the projects had documented the short-comings in their managerial structures and approached these initiatives as an opportunity to impact client services and organizational culture. Now, in the third year of this process, the words of Rosabeth Kanter in Challenge of Organizational Change ring particularly true: "The sad fact is that, almost universally, organizations change as little as they must, rather than as much as they should" (1992, p. 4).

A clear advantage that the initiatives described in this issue had is that they all commenced with some mandated research design in place and a generally agreed upon approach to evidence-based practice. The operational construct used draws on Baker's definition from the Social Work Dictionary (1995) which includes the elements of research as both a practice and problem-solving tool, systematic data collection to monitor intervention, specifying problems, techniques and outcomes in measurable terms and regularly evaluating the effectiveness of interventions used. The ultimate goal of evidence-based practice is interventions for which there is consistent scientific evidence showing that they improve client outcomes (Drake et al., 2001). Each project was constructed to test a different model of clinical supervision and track its impact on client outcomes. The articles in this issue attest to the struggles that the

---

[Haworth co-indexing entry note]: "Foreword." Jones, Jenny L., and Paul Sundet. Co-published simultaneously in *Journal of Evidence-Based Social Work* (The Haworth Press, Inc.) Vol. 4, No. 3/4, 2007, pp. xxi-xxiii; and: *Developing an Empirically Based Practice Initiative: A Case Study in CPS Supervision* (ed: Jenny L. Jones, and Paul Sundet) The Haworth Press, Inc., 2007, pp. xiii-xv. Single or multiple copies of this article are available for a fee from The Haworth Document Delivery Service [1-800-HAWORTH 9:00 a.m. - 5:00 p.m. (EST). E-mail address: docdelivery@haworthpress.com].

Available online at http://jebsw.haworthpress.com

doi:10.1300/J394v04n03

project staffs have had to live up to that ideal as well as some of the notable successes that have been achieved with the very modest resources available.

And in this regard the offering here are exemplary of the state of such practice in the field of child welfare. A quick review of the Cochrane and Campbell Collections yields scant returns on the subject despite the mandates contained in the Adoption and Safe Families Act of 1997. The federal Child and Family Service Review process, while markedly flawed from a methodological standpoint, has never-the-less given impetus to increased efforts within the states and has abetted the rise of important initiatives such as the California Clearinghouse, the Children and Family Research Center at University of Illinois at Urbana/Champaign, the University of Kansas' Results Oriented Management in Child Welfare program and the oversight structure for these programs, Southern Regional Quality Improvement Center, University of Kentucky (SR-QIC).

While the barriers to the systematic research required for solid evidence-based practice are many, three categories stand out in these projects. First is the obvious paucity of both financial and technical resources. Internal agency research components are meager and their focus is primarily on management information systems to meet mandated fiscal and programmatic requirements. Scant attention is paid to assessing causal or even correlational relationships. With limited funds, often little internal technical expertise, and pressing competition for budget share with essential line activities, "research" is frequently viewed as a luxury that can or must be dispensed with in light of other priorities. A second barrier category we have chosen to label contextual concerns. Various professional organizations (besides the Cochrane/Campbell noted above) have promulgated criteria for assessing whether a program or intervention has been sufficiently empirically validated to merit being termed efficacious or effective. Included in that number are the National Institutes of Health, the National Science Foundation and most recently the Society for Prevention Research's Standards of Evidence (Flay, 2004). The conditions posited for validity and reliability in these documents are almost totally foreign to practitioners in the typical child welfare system. Longitudinal studies with long-term follow-up are rare at best. Program stability over the life of an intervention is difficult to maintain in the ever-changing public sector. Random assignment of participants is fraught with political pitfalls and systematic control of potential contaminants assumes administrative aegis beyond the sway of most researchers. Programs showing any preliminary promise are frequently rolled-out for broad dissemination before their maturity and prior to adequate comparison analyses have been completed. The pristine conditions for efficacy testing give way to the compromises of "real-world" conditions, a bargaining process in which the research component is often holding the short stack of chips. The third category of constraint to systematic research is ideological. Much of social work practice is based on values and nowhere is that more evident than in child welfare where core issues such as the operational definitions of well-being and safety are continually debated and the relative weight of child and parental rights remains a matter of contention. In this environment there is a strong tradition of reliance on practitioner judgment as the proximate guide for action. Reliance is placed on personal experience rather than external evidence. The value continually cited is "individualization" where primacy is placed on the uniqueness of each case situation and that following general rules derived from research does not produce the best outcomes. Tradition and intuition become the markers for practice rather than evidence derived through scientific method.

All of these elements have impacted the research that has and is being conducted in these training and demonstration projects. And the almost amazing outcome is that despite formidable barriers, quality research is being conducted and it is leading to evidence-based changes in agency policy and practices in all four jurisdictions. The Children's Bureau and the SR-QIC are to be commended for demanding rigor in design and execution of both formative and summative evaluation. And we applaud the efforts of our colleagues to remain true to the original intent of model testing. We would hasten to add that these empirically-based interventions have not been a panacea which made every issue go away. But what they have done is help these organizations think rationally about the issues they encounter and the most effective and efficient means of addressing them. It has been a way of surfacing and then answering questions. Thus, it has been an important beginning.

Jenny L. Jones, PhD
Paul Sundet, PhD

REFERENCES

Baker, R.L. (2004). Social Work Dictionary. Washington, DC: NASW Press.

Drake, R., Goldman, H., Leff, H., Lehman, A., Dixon, L., Mueser, K., and Torrey,W. (2001). Implementing evidence-based practice in routine mental health service settings. Psychiatric Services, 52:179-182.

Flay, B. (2004). Standards of Evidence. Falls Church, VA: Society for Prevention Research.

Kanter, Rosabeth M. (1992). Challenge of Organizational Change. New York: Free Press.

Introduction

Among the various fields of social work practice there is, perhaps, none in which the dearth of evidence-based practice is as notable as in child protective services. By comparison to the allied discipline of early child development, the social work literature is meager indeed. Numerous explanations have been put forward to account for the deficits ranging from emphasis on ritualistic case counting to the paucity of the necessary ancillary resources in child welfare agencies to the inherent nature of the work and its confounding variables. However, none of these sufficiently excuse the profession from its obligation to systematically examine the tenets of practice. It is, therefore, with enthusiasm that we welcome the increased emphasis that is currently being place on formal research and evaluation in this critical field.

This volume is devoted to one notable effort to add to the growing body of scientific literature in this arena. All of the articles arise from a three year training/demonstration project for child welfare supervisors in four southeastern states. Children's Bureau, in a departure from past practices, has attempted to decentralize decision-making in these pilots while, concurrently, setting higher standards for evidence-based practice. Brodowski and her associates detail this initiative from the federal perspective while Collins-Camargo discusses its operational implications at the SE Regional Quality Improvement level. She cogently details the issues of providing technical research assistance to child welfare agencies and the complexities of cross-site evaluation with disparate political jurisdictions. Building on this premise, Ellett examines the linkage between perceived self-efficacy, staff retention and development of instrumentation that can be used to measure organizational culture. Secondary traumatic stress and its impact on front-line workers is studied by Bride, Jones and MacMaster suggesting that issues of peer support

[Haworth co-indexing entry note]: "Introduction." Wodarski, John. Co-published simultaneously in the *Journal of Evidence-Based Social Work* (The Haworth Press, Inc.) Vol. 4, No. 3/4, 2007, pp. 1-2; and: *Developing an Empirically Based Practice Inititative: A Case Study in CPS Supervision* (ed: Jenny L. Jones, and Paul Sundet) The Haworth Press, 2007, pp. 1-2. Single or multiple copies of this article are available for a fee from The Haworth Document Delivery Service [1-800-HAWORTH, 9:00 a.m. - 5:00 p.m. (EST). E-mail address: docdelivery@haworthpress.com].

Available online at http://jebsw.haworthpress.com

doi:10.1300/J394v04n03_01

and manageable caseload size are critical elements impacting stress levels. The Arkansas state project (Murphy and Goodson) tackles the thorny issue of limitations in standardized instruments in an experimental design when applied to highly idiosyncratic interventions and appeals for a balance of qualitative and quantitative measures. The Tennessee Project, like the other four states involved in this effort has worked to enhance clinical decision-making skills among supervisors. Jones, Washington, and Steppe address the concerns regarding clinical decision-making and present a framework that can be used to facilitate this process. All fifty states have had difficulty in meeting the outcome based federal standards (CSFR) in child welfare and Shackelford, Harper, Sullivan and Edwards describe how enlisting the Mississippi child welfare supervisors in a systematic case review process has improved documented outcomes despite administrative hurdles.

While the business industry has used the 360-degree evaluation process to develop staff, human services organizations have been slow to adopt this technology. Kelly and Sundet document its application to child welfare supervision and workers' changes in perceived effectiveness of their superiors when systematic individual development plans are instituted. Steppe and Jones bring the dual perspective of a top agency administrator and an academic to discussion of the constraints that agency and political realities place on multi-year research designs and offer suggestions for planners of such efforts. Finally, Sundet and Kelly revisit the classic social work literature to examine how the specific expertise of the academy and the service agency can be melded into research and demonstration efforts that provide empirical evidence for policy decisions and program adoption.

These articles provide a beginning in examining issues pertaining to child welfare supervision and demonstrate that research methodology can be mated to staff training to enhance the quality of evidence-based practice in this field. The editors Feit, Wodarski, and Dulmus appreciate the contributions from the field of child welfare and would like to acknowledge the guest editors (Jones and Sundet) for their contributions in the development of this special edition.

John Wodarski, PhD
Editor

existing knowledge and evidence gleaned from the research and practice to guide policy, funding, and, ultimately, program practice.

Despite the growing body of knowledge in child abuse and neglect and child welfare, the field is still starved for information on what works. The existing research points to the fact that there are no easy answers to the many layers of questions. There is also an inherent challenge in balancing the need to rapidly secure information about new programs and practices with the need to allow time for programs to mature and for rigorous evaluations to be conducted. Outcome evaluations ultimately may or may not support the early enthusiasm that often accompanies new programs. While there may be concerns about prematurely disseminating information about unproven programs or practices, waiting for final evaluation findings may further frustrate the needs of the field for new information that may help them improve their policies and practices.

There is general agreement that the field needs to move beyond the identification of model programs or model program components. The field is now asking questions and seeking answers about more specific issues such as: what works best for whom, and in what situations. Other emerging research interests include:

- How does one create agency cultures that are receptive to evidence, evidence-based practice, and sustainable change?
- Transferring and replicating programs: How can you truly replicate a program with high fidelity from another setting?
- Translating programs: Can an organization make adaptations to a model program and maintain the positive outcomes achieved in the original model?
- What does it really take to implement these "successful" programs?
- How can we sustain successful programs?
- Dissemination: How can we share the information and lessons learned in a meaningful way?

Knowledge development and knowledge management incorporate these activities–identify, transfer, translate, sustain, and disseminate.

One approach to answering these questions is described in this article. It provides an overview of the Children's Bureau discretionary grant programs; a discussion of the Bureau's approach to grant-making towards knowledge development and knowledge management; and a review of the specific strategies that the Bureau is undertaking to promote and support this philosophy. The article will also provide two examples of how this concept has been implemented through specific grant clusters: the Quality Improvement Centers on Child Protective Services and Adoption, and the Replications of a Demonstrated Effective Prevention Program (a.k.a. Family Connections Prevention Replications). The article will conclude with a discussion about the next steps for the Children's Bureau and its continued efforts to move the field of child welfare forward, generate knowledge, and disseminate information that can truly inform policy and practice to improve outcomes for children and their families.

CHILDREN'S BUREAU DISCRETIONARY GRANT PROGRAMS

Each year, the Children's Bureau, Administration for Children and Families, U.S. Department of Health and Human Services, invests approximately $110 million dollars in building the knowledge base for child abuse and neglect and child welfare services. These discretionary activities fund a variety of research and demonstration grants, training and technical assistance cooperative agreements, and multi-year research contracts. As part of this effort, the Children's Bureau manages more than 200 grants, cooperative agreements, contracts, and interagency agreements, with awards ranging from $100,000 to several million dollars per year, averaging about $300,000 per year for research and service demonstration projects. Each project is testing a specific research hypothesis or service model, covering a wide range of topics related to child maltreatment, child protective services, child welfare, adoption, and child abuse and neglect prevention, treatment, and intervention (U.S. Department of Health and Human Services, 2005).

As the primary Federal agency with responsibility for overseeing child welfare and child abuse and neglect funding for State agencies, the Children's Bureau has been striving to move the field of child welfare towards more evidence-based practice by disseminating the knowledge gained through our discretionary grant activities. Within the parameters of legislative authority, discretionary grants permit the Federal government, to identify a range of priority areas to be supported by the funding. Some of the current discretionary grant programs include:

- The **Child Abuse Prevention & Treatment Act Research and Demonstration Projects** support research on the causes, prevention, and treatment of child abuse and neglect; demonstration programs to identify the best means of preventing maltreatment and treating troubled families; and the development and implementation of training programs.

- The **Adoption Opportunities Program** supports projects, which aim to eliminate barriers to adoption and help to find permanent families for children who would benefit by adoption, particularly children with special needs.
- The **Abandoned Infants Assistance program** provides funding for the development of comprehensive service programs to infants and their families to demonstrate strategies to: identify and address needs of abandoned infants, especially those with AIDS.
- The **Promoting Safe and Stable Families program** provides funding for research, evaluation and technical assistance related to the four priority funding areas outlined in the legislation: family support, family preservation, time-limited family reunification services, and services to promote and support adoptions. These services are primarily aimed at preventing the risk of abuse and promoting nurturing families, assisting families at risk of having a child removed from their home, promoting the timely return of a child to his/her home, and if returning home is not an option, placement of a child in a permanent setting with services that support the family.
- The **Child Welfare Services Training program** upgrades the skills and qualifications of child welfare workers through their participation, full-time or part-time, in programs focused specifically on child welfare services. Discretionary grants are awarded to public and private non-profit institutions of higher learning to develop and improve education/training programs and resources for child welfare service providers.
- The **Infant Adoption Awareness Training Program** (IAATP) provides support for developing and implementing new training curriculum and evaluating and adapting existing IAATP training programs and/or curricula to train designated staff of eligible health centers in providing adoption information and referrals to pregnant women on an equal basis with all other courses of action included in nondirective counseling to pregnant women.

Discretionary Grant Program Philosophical Principles

Child welfare legislation has always fostered the concept of using discretionary grants for promoting knowledge development. However, in previous years, discretionary grants had focused more on providing funds to augment local resources for desperately needed service delivery. The Federal funding provided an opportunity to support interesting programs and innovative strategies that met identified needs. These projects may or may not have included an evaluation of the project or significant planning for institutionalizing change and sustaining successful programs when Federal funding ended. Since the early 1990s, the Children's Bureau has been making a concerted effort to maximize the benefits of its limited discretionary grant funds by investing them in knowledge development–finding out what works so child welfare programs can be more effective.

Today, grants are viewed as investments in knowledge by the Federal government and the Bureau has been placing higher standards and expectations on applicants and grantees. We are very much interested in, and require that knowledge be gained from our research and demonstration projects. We want to know everything about the processes, the outcomes and the lessons learned from our various projects. We believe that this focus on knowledge is the best way to gain a sound return on the financial investment of the grant award. In addition, we are actively finding ways to use the information and to disseminate the findings in more strategic ways. Grantees are now being told directly that we are funding research and demonstration projects and that our discretionary grants are not meant only to fund services. Although a demonstration project may include the provision of services, the funds are meant to support the piloting of the concept (a.k.a. the experiment) and not meant for sustained funding. Although most grantees are open to this concept, old habits die hard and some programs continue to view their Federal grant as support for their own existing programs. These programs tend to view the research and evaluation aspects of their projects as less important than the services they provide.

The Children's Bureau's philosophical shift echoes a larger movement towards demonstrating outcomes and exercising accountability within Federal government programs. This has been a guiding principle for over a decade since the passage of the Government Results and Performance Act of 1993, which is an effort to systematically hold Federal agencies accountable for achieving program results. It is also an attempt to improve Federal program effectiveness and public accountability by promoting a new focus on results, service quality, and customer satisfaction. More recently, the Office of Management and Budget developed a Program Assessment Rating Tool (PART) in 2002 as a way to rate government programs on their effectiveness. The PART evaluation reviews four critical areas in the assessment:

purpose and design, strategic planning, management, and results and accountability. Each section is scored and programs receive ratings from ineffective to effective. Despite the inherent difficulties in rating complex Federal programs and funding streams in this manner, both GPRA and PART are processes by which the Federal government is seeking information to justify the effectiveness and impact of funds for particular programs and activities. In addition, the scarce dollars available to support programs and agencies in child welfare have resulted in policy makers and administrators being much more selective and insistent that funding go to support programs and strategies that have demonstrated positive results and are likely to have direct national, state or local applicability.

The child welfare field has been moving in this direction as well. The Adoption and Safe Families Act of 1997 and the resulting regulations hold States accountable for services to at-risk children and children in foster care through the Child and Families Services Reviews, which are a results-oriented approach in Federal monitoring of state child welfare programs. Under this Federal review process, states are assessed on the quality of services provided to, and outcome results for, at-risk children, for the first time. States receiving poor reviews will be given the opportunity to undertake corrective action plans. If standards are not met within certain time periods, States may also be subject to tough new penalties. Despite the threat of penalties, the Children's Bureau is striving to work in partnership with the States to improve outcomes for children and families.

Federal legislation and current political and social landscapes have shaped the way in which the Children's Bureau now manages our discretionary grants program and how we respond to our different constituencies. Our target population is comprised of both a vertical and a horizontal audience. The vertical audience refers to the policy makers, legislators, and administrators who we hope will use the knowledge gained from research to guide their decision-making. The horizontal audience refers to the direct program and practice staff that need and use information from the research to guide their practice in working with families. Both audiences are equally important, but each requires a different approach and will need different types of knowledge and information. Prior to the reorganization of the Children's Bureau in 1996, the National Center on Child Abuse and Neglect was more actively involved in information dissemination efforts and developed multiple publications on specific topics related to child maltreatment. The National Clearinghouse on Child Abuse and Neglect Information was also undertaking its own efforts to disseminate knowledge to the field. However, the Bureau has been greatly dependent on the grantees themselves to horizontally disseminate the information through journal publications and conference presentations. In the last few years, we realized that we needed to take a more active role in that dissemination process as well. There is a Federal responsibility to bridge the gap that continues to exist between the research our tax dollars fund and the practice of child welfare that also depends on Federal, State and local funds.

As part of this effort, the Children's Bureau is beginning to explore strategies for the management of the knowledge that exits as a product of the grants that we are funding–as well as the knowledge from other research that is available. Knowledge management is a concept that has its origins in the business and information technology sectors. The concept of finding ways to organize, have accessible, and use existing data and information has direct applicability to the knowledge management efforts that the Children's Bureau, and other Federal agencies have embarked on. At its core, knowledge management is simply the process of getting the right information to the people who need it, when they need it, in a form that is useful to them. A number of Federal agencies and other private organizations have launched knowledge management efforts. These include the Substance Abuse and Mental Health Services Administration (SAMHSA) National Registry of Effective Programs, Office of Juvenile Justice and Delinquency Prevention (OJJDP) Blueprints for Violence Prevention, the Office of Victim's of Crime (OVC) Treatment Guidelines, the Centers for Disease Control (CDC) Community Guides, Ewing M. Kaufman Foundation's Best Practices in Child Welfare, the Promising Practices Network, and Child Welfare League of America's R2P (Research to Practice) Initiative, which are all vehicles for organizing the best available research and knowledge on a variety or programs and making that information available to the field.

THE DISCRETIONARY GRANT CYCLE AS A MEANS FOR KNOWLEDGE DEVELOPMENT

Our discretionary grant cycle is the mechanism by which we operationalize our philosophy around knowledge development and our efforts to bridge the gap from research to practice by supporting research translation with our vertical and horizontal audiences. The starting point is the funding announcement phase. During this phase the Bureau identifies knowledge gaps, generates ideas for new funding announcements and writes announcements for the availability of funds. This first planning phase begins with a review of the relevant statutory language to identify areas that need to be funded according to the requirements of the legislation. A variety of other data sources are also taken into consideration: Administration priorities, the lessons learned from previous grant projects, research and lessons learned from the field, and more recently, the results of the Child and Family Services Reviews. In this way, the announcements are developed and written using the rich body of knowledge that is available. Thus, the announcements both lead and seed innovation.

After the announcements are written and issued, and applications are received from the field, the next phase is the grant review process. The Bureau, like other Federal agencies, utilizes a peer review process which brings together researchers, practitioners, and program administrators working in child abuse and neglect, adoption, foster care, and child welfare for an in-person, intensive grant review process. After the review panels review and score the applications, the applications are ranked according to scores. Bureau staff provides input and works with our administrators and political leadership to finalize funding decisions and award the grants.

Once the grant awards are made, the next phase focuses on monitoring implementation and progress. During this period, the Federal Project Officers work with their respective grantees, through a variety of activities to monitor and review program progress. Semi-annual written reports are required of every grantee, as well as a final report submitted at the end of the grant period. The information provided through these reports is a critical resource for the Bureau's knowledge development activity. In addition, grantees are required to disseminate the information from their projects to a wide audience. To support these efforts, the Bureau also works with grantees to find ways to share lessons learned (i.e., promote knowledge development and knowledge management) all along the way so that the information will be made available sooner than the end of the grant period.

STRATEGIES TO PROMOTE KNOWLEDGE DEVELOPMENT

The Bureau has implemented a number of specific strategies over the last several years to infuse our knowledge development philosophy into our discretionary grant programs. These strategies fall into three broad categories: (1) requirements for grant applicants; (2) post award grant monitoring; and (3) information dissemination and research translation.

Requirements for Grant Applicants

All new funding announcements include a general requirement that applicants include a logic model as part of their application. A logic model is a tool that presents the conceptual framework for a proposed project and explains the linkages among program elements and intended outcomes. While there are many versions of the logic model, they generally summarize the logical connections among the needs that are the focus of the project, project goals and objectives, the target population, project inputs (resources), the proposed activities/processes/outputs directed toward the target population, the expected short- and long-term outcomes the initiative is designed to achieve, and the evaluation plan for measuring the extent to which proposed processes and outcomes actually occur.

We have also required that grantees allocate 10-15% of their proposed budget to an evaluation of their funded project, ideally using an external evaluator. Announcements from the last two years have included standardized language that grantees must work with any potential national evaluation of the project as well. Applicants are asked to describe their program evaluation plans in detail. Specific evaluation criteria are included so reviewers can rate the quality of the applications' evaluation plans. Finally, we have also included language that grantees must seek the appropriate institutional review of human subject protections for the proposed projects. Since we view the discretionary grants as knowledge generating activities, we have been encouraging our grantees to follow appropriate procedures to protect the privacy of the program participants and ensure the confidentiality of the information about them. Applicants planning to gather data from individual participants, as opposed to system or program level data, are asked specifically to describe their plans regarding Institutional Review Board (IRB) review.

Post-Award Grant Monitoring

Once the grant is awarded, Federal Project Officers and Grant Specialists work closely with their grantees to monitor the grant and provide technical assistance and support on the requirements of the grant. There are two mechanisms by which the Bureau awards discretionary funding: grants and cooperative agreements. The traditional grant provides funding to the grantee for the idea they proposed to advance the field with typically less government oversight. A cooperative agreement is another type of grant in which substantial Federal involvement is anticipated. A cooperative agreement clearly defines the respective responsibilities of the Children's Bureau and the grantee prior to the award. The Children's Bureau anticipates that our involvement will produce programmatic benefits to the recipient otherwise unavailable to them for carrying out the project. Recently, more grants are being awarded as cooperative agreements, which reflect the Bureau's greater interest in participating in the overall direction setting and management for particular sets of grantees or grant clusters (i.e., a cohort of grants for one topic area all of whom have responded to the same grant announcement).

Each grantee is required to attend an annual meeting hosted by the Children's Bureau. Over the last three years, the Children's Bureau has also required attendance at an early a kick-off meeting in Washington, DC within 90 days of the grant award. The Federal staff and grantees have reported that the early meetings are critical since they provide an opportunity to meet the Federal Project Officers in person and also to hear about the vision and goals that the Bureau has for the grant cluster. It is also an opportunity to answer initial questions and provide a way for grantees to begin developing a peer network.

The Bureau has been very interested in fostering the development of local research networks. We believe that local networks provide easy access to informational resources, support a community-responsibility approach to solving child welfare problems, and may have a better understanding of local contexts that impact research and service delivery. To foster ongoing communication, the Bureau has used technology to foster the establishment of virtual learning communities. This is most evident through the establishment of list serves for specific grantee clusters. The list serves provide an opportunity for communication with the Federal Project Officers and across grantees throughout the year. The Children's Bureau is also researching the use of discussion boards and other ways that online communication can be further enhanced by available technology. Some Federal Project Officers, particularly those with cooperative agreements, schedule a monthly call for all the projects in a grant cluster as a way to monitor progress and create a peer network, as well as address specific issues related to the implementation of the project. These calls have been an opportunity to share lessons learned with other projects and further strengthen the peer network across like projects.

A key component of providing additional support to grantees is through a contract that the Children's Bureau has with James Bell Associates (JBA) to provide technical assistance to the grantees regarding project evaluation. JBA is available to help grantees develop logic models, evaluation plans (if there is no evaluator available), and provide workshops for the grantees on a variety of topics. JBA conducts site visits to the grantees, prepares summary profiles for each of the grantees, and writes evaluation synthesis reports on the findings from the grantees' reports. More recently, JBA has developed generic and more specific 6-month progress and final report templates for certain grantee clusters, when requested by the Project Officer. JBA is available to assist grantees to become better prepared in the event the Bureau is able to conduct a national cross-site evaluation.

JBA has provided evaluation technical assistance to the grantees since 1998. When the contract first began, many grantees were uncomfortable with the expectations about an evaluation and were reluctant to access the technical assistance available. More recently, JBA has noted a considerable increase in grantees' interest both in conducting their own evaluations and in learning more from other grantees' evaluations. It is possible that the increased emphasis on evaluation on the part of the Children's Bureau has helped change the attitudes of the grantees toward evaluation. Also, the Children's Bureau has provided JBA with a forum to discuss evaluation issues with grantees at the orientation meetings for new grantees. Reviewing logic models and evaluation plans with grantees at the start of their projects has helped create a positive environment for grantees to seek assistance. It has also provided an opportunity for grantees within the same cluster to consider common evaluation approaches and measures. Although JBA continues to provide individualized assistance to grantees, efforts to provide assistance to grantees as a cluster have increased, thereby strengthening the feasibility of ultimately synthesizing findings across projects.

Information Dissemination and Research Translation

Finally, the Children's Bureau is committed to disseminating the knowledge gained from our discretionary grants in a more purposeful and planful way. The Bureau's National Clearinghouses on Child Abuse and Neglect Information and Adoption are the gateway for information for the broader child welfare community. We have been working closely with the Clearinghouse to disseminate the knowledge from our discretionary grants in a much more comprehensive, yet user-friendly manner. Our focus on this activity was reinforced by Congress during the reauthorization of the Child Abuse Prevention and Treatment Act (CAPTA), in 2003, which included language directing the Clearinghouse "to maintain, collect, and disseminate information on all effective programs, especially those showing promise of success with respect to the prevention, assessment, identification, and treatment of child abuse and neglect and hold promise for broad scale implementation and replication." The Bureau is very interested in disseminating information that would be of interest to the field in general, especially that gleaned from funded projects. As part of this process, over the last few years, the Clearinghouse has been developing synthesis reports of the findings from specific grantee clusters. Some recent syntheses that have been disseminated include those addressing the topics of child neglect prevention, treatment and intervention; decision making in unsubstantiated Child Protective Services cases; and school-based child maltreatment programs. These syntheses reports are based on the final reports from the grantees and highlight the most relevant information that professionals in the field are likely to be most interested in, in the most user-friendly, succinct, straightforward way. Other new products being developed by the Clearinghouse include "Practice Briefs" that take information in the research synthesis and develop a more concise written document especially for practitioners. The Practice Brief presents the information in ways that clearly translate the research findings to applications directly to their practice. Finally, the Clearinghouse has recently updated its website to ensure that information is more accessible to anyone seeking this information.

THE QUALITY IMPROVEMENT CENTERS (QICs) ON CPS AND ADOPTION

In fiscal year 2001, under the Adoption Opportunities Program and the Child Abuse and Prevention and Treatment Act Program, the Children's Bureau awarded cooperative agreements to organizations to implement regional Quality Improvement Centers (QICs) in the areas of child protective services (CPS) and adoption. The QICs represent a new approach to Children's Bureau grant making and hold promise as a vehicle for supporting a more regionalized approach to building the evidence base in child welfare. The purpose of the QICs is to promote knowledge development with the overarching goal of improving child welfare services. The QICs represent an experiment by the Children's Bureau to examine the feasibility and benefits of increasing regional involvement in designing and managing research and demonstration efforts. In addition, each QIC is required to disseminate the findings of their activities throughout their region and nationally (U.S. Department of Health and Human Services, 2001).

The QICs are charged with planning and implementing research or demonstration grants on topics the QICs selected with input from individual regional advisory groups with Federal approval. The QICs established their regional advisory groups, identified a general area of interest, and undertook a needs assessment activity to collect data and identify a specific topic during the first year. They are each funding, monitoring, supporting and evaluating three or four research and demonstration projects in their region during years 2 through 4 and disseminating findings during year 5. Each QIC had issued a Request for Applications for projects on their chosen topic area. Each required that applicants include a plan for evaluating their demonstration project in their proposal.

There is also a national evaluation of the QIC model being conducting by James Bell Associates. Preliminary data from the QIC's local grantees indicate that there is a significant need for training and technical assistance on evaluation and building capacity of organizations to implement their planned interventions. The QICs provided technical assistance to potential applicants during the application process and have continued to provide assistance after the local grants were awarded. The local grantees have noted that the QICs have provided them with a level of technical assistance that they had not previously received from other funding sources.

Local grantees have also noted that the QICs have been very responsive to these needs, successfully creating a local resource network in their regions for individual project support. Though, at first blush, the QIC may appear to create an additional level of bureaucracy, the design supports the philosophical notion of moving resource management closer to the local level, where better understanding of the research context is more likely to create lasting partnerships for seeking solutions to local problems and applying these solutions on a community level. Like some of the clusters of Federal discretionary grantees, the QICs' local grantees appear to particularly appreciate the opportunities the QICs have provided to share information with the other grantees in their region and to develop plans to share information from each other's programs.

Through their efforts to date, the QICs succeeded in serving as a vehicle for funding, managing and providing assistance to a group of regionally dispersed grantees. The successes of the QICs include the following:

- All local grantees fully implemented their demonstrations.
- All local grantees received extensive technical assistance that they needed on a wide range of topics.

- All of the local grantees employed third-party evaluators to conduct an evaluation and participate in the development of the cross-site evaluation plans.
- All QICs established collaborative networks among the Advisory Group members and local grantees as well as other relevant stakeholders.
- All QICs began dissemination about their efforts. QICs made joint and individual presentations at national conferences. They also made presentations in collaboration with their local grantees. QICs also held forums, wrote journal articles and established websites to communicate their findings with others in the child welfare and adoption fields.
- Two of the QICs received additional grants on topics related to their initial research plans.
- All QICs began to work with their grantees to consider ways of sustaining their efforts after the current grant period ends.

While it is still too soon to make a definitive assessment of the QICs, evidence to date suggests that they present a promising vehicle for the development and dissemination of evidence-based practice and for managing and assisting a set of local grantees in conducting demonstration projects on a common topic.

REPLICATIONS OF A DEMONSTRATED EFFECTIVE PREVENTION PROGRAM

The Preventions Replications cluster is another specific example of the way in which the knowledge development philosophy has been infused into the grantees project and cross-site involvement. In 2003, the Children's Bureau released the report, *Emerging Practices in the Prevention of Child Abuse and Neglect*, which highlighted effective and innovation prevention programs selected through a national nomination process. The report also provided a literature review regarding the types of prevention programs that exist today and a review of the research on their effectiveness. Through this process, the Family Connections program, based at the University of Maryland in Baltimore, was the only program designated as "demonstrated effective" in showing positive outcomes in the prevention of child abuse and neglect. Family Connections is a community-based neglect prevention program targeting at-risk families with children between the ages of 5 and 11. As a follow-up to the *Emerging Practices* report, in FY2003 the Children's Bureau issued a funding announcement to provide financial support to replicate and evaluate critical components of programs that have been previously demonstrated to be successful at preventing or reducing the risk of child maltreatment, testing their effectiveness in other settings. The projects funded under this priority area were to incorporate features and components that hold promise for contributing to an expansion of the knowledge base about effective strategies in child abuse and neglect prevention. The eight projects selected for funding all proposed to replicate critical components of the Family Connections (FC) program.

The replication projects were awarded as cooperative agreements between the grantee and the Children's Bureau, allowing for considerable input, on a continuing basis, by the Bureau. Each project was awarded both planning and implementation funds. At the end of the planning phase (11 months), each project developed and submitted for Children's Bureau approval, an implementation plan for their replication project. Each project has made revisions to their implementation plan based on Children's Bureau input and was given approval to move forward. Each project will be expected, during the implementation phase (1 month plus 4 years), to manage, administer the program, monitor and evaluate the replication projects. The evaluation design must include plans for a cost-analysis of the project. All projects are currently in their first year of implementation, which began October 2004.

With technical assistance and support from James Bell Associates, the National Center for Injury Control and Prevention at the Centers for Disease Control, and the National Data Archive on Child Abuse and Neglect, the following has been accomplished by this grantee cluster:

- Identified and agreed upon the Family Connections fidelity criteria which outline the critical components of the model;
- Identified and agreed upon cross-site outcome measures and instruments in the domains of risk and protective factors, and child safety and well-being;
- Identified and agreed upon cross-site data elements to be submitted to the National Data Archive on Child Abuse and Neglect;
- Identified and agreed upon cross-site cost analysis data elements for the Pre-Implementation and Implementation phases of the project;
- Agreed upon a common framework for the local evaluations which include informed consent and random assignment to treatment and control groups, and a plan for conducting intent to treat analysis as part of their evaluation plans.

Throughout every discussion, this cluster of projects viewed themselves as part of a larger network of grantees all working towards advancing the state of the art in prevention science.

FUTURE DIRECTIONS

As we continue to issue new funding announcements and receive the reports from the Bureau's ongoing research and demonstration projects, we must continue to examine how these findings contribute to the knowledge base in child welfare. It will be important to examine and continually refine the criteria we use to identify what we mean by knowledge itself. We will need to distinguish between useful knowledge that must be information the Bureau and Clearinghouses will "push out"–and other useful information that does not need to be shared widely, but should be available to those who seek it or want to "pull" it out. We also need to examine what information is the most useful for certain groups of people and professionals. These questions will most likely be different depending on the target audience. We will need to tailor our information dissemination efforts using both push and pull activities to satisfy both the vertical and horizontal audiences.

We plan to continually work with our Clearinghouse and our constituents to insure that people have access to the information and the research when they most need it, in a format that is most useful for their purposes. Other Federal agencies are also working along similar lines. SAMSHA has implemented an initiative called "science to service." CDC has presented about the concept of "translational research." Other Federal agencies are in the same situation, maximizing the Federal investment by meeting the need to share the lessons learned from our funding projects with the field. We will continue to work to in partnership with other federal agencies, nongovernmental entities, and the research and practice communities to inform and move the field of child welfare towards true evidence-based policies, programs and practice.

REFERENCES

Chadwick Center on Children and Families. (2004). *Closing the quality chasm in child abuse treatment: Identifying and disseminating best practices*. San Diego, CA: Author.

Chaffin, M. & Friedlich, B. (2004). Evidence-based treatments in child abuse and neglect. *Child and Youth Services Review, 26*, 1097-1113.

Hensler, D., Wilson, C. & Sadler, D. (2003). *Closing the Quality Chasm in Child Abuse Treatment: Identifying and Disseminating Best Practices. The Findings from the Kaufman Best Practices Project.* (website).

Schinke, S., Brounstein, P. & Gardner S. *Science-Based Prevention Programs and Principles, 2002.* DHHS Pub. No. (SMA) 03-3764. Rockville, MD: Center for Substance Abuse Prevention, Substance Abuse and Mental Health Services Administration, 2002.

U.S. Department of Justice, Office of Justice Programs, Office of Juvenile Justice and Delinquency Prevention (OJJDP). (2004). *Blueprints for Violence Prevention.* Washington, DC: U.S. Government Printing Office.

U.S. Department of Health and Human Services (DHHS), Administration for Children and Families, Children's Bureau. (2001). *Application Package to Request Financial Assistance FY 2001.* Washington, DC: U.S. Government Printing Office.

U.S. Department of Health and Human Services (DHHS), Administration for Children and Families, Children's Bureau. (2005). Based on information provided by budget officer.

U.S. Department of Health and Human Services (DHHS), Administration for Children and Families, Children's Bureau. (2003). Closing Plenary Session–Annual Meeting of States and Tribes, January 29, 2003, Comments by Jerry Milner. *http://www.acf.hhs.gov/programs/cb/cwrp/changing_culture.htm*

Wilson, C. (2004). Exploring alternative strategies to diffusion of best practice. Presentation at the Children's Bureau Evidence-Based Child Welfare Conference, Washington, DC, July 2004.

doi:10.1300/J394v04n03_02

Administering Research and Demonstration Projects Aimed at Promoting Evidence-Based Practice in Child Welfare: Challenges and Rewards

Crystal Collins-Camargo, MSW, ABD

SUMMARY. The Southern Regional Quality Improvement Center for Child Protection, funded by the Children's Bureau is administering research and demonstration projects in public child welfare agencies in four states to test models of structured clinical supervision in achieving organizational, social worker and client outcomes. These projects represent an attempt to promote evidence-based practice in the public agency. These projects are discussed within the context of the status of evidence-based practice in social work. The university has experienced number of challenges in provided technical assistance and conducting the cross-site evaluation of these projects which may be of interest to others attempting to foster evidence-based practice in this type of environment.

Crystal Collins-Camargo is Clinical Assistant Professor, University of Kentucky College of Social Work, 1 Quality Street, Suite 700, Lexington, KY 40507.

[Haworth co-indexing entry note]: "Administering Research and Demonstration Projects Aimed at Promoting Evidence-Based Practice in Child Welfare: Challenges and Rewards." Collins-Camargo, Crystal. Co-published simultaneously in the *Journal of Evidence-Based Social Work* (The Haworth Press, Inc.) Vol. 4, No. 3/4, 2007, pp. 21-38; and: *Developing an Empirically Based Practice Inititative: A Case Study in CPS Supervision* (ed: Jenny L. Jones, and Paul Sundet) The Haworth Press, 2007, pp. 21-38. Single or multiple copies of this article are available for a fee from The Haworth Document Delivery Service [1-800-HAWORTH, 9:00 a.m. - 5:00 p.m. (EST). E-mail address: docdelivery@haworthpress.com].

Available online at http://jebsw.haworthpress.com

doi:10.1300/J394v04n03_03

These challenges, as well as promising solutions, are detailed in this article.
doi:10.1300/J394v04n03_03 *[Article copies available for a fee from The Haworth Document Delivery Service: 1-800-HAWORTH. E-mail address: <docdelivery@haworthpress.com> Website: <http://www.HaworthPress.com>*

KEYWORDS. Evidence-based practice, child welfare, social work, technical assistance

INTRODUCTION

Recent years have seen the call for child welfare agencies and their employees to be held responsible for evaluating the effectiveness of their services in achieving appropriate outcomes for children and families (Waldfogel, 1998; Waldfogel, 2000a). Research into the ability of the public child protection system to achieve its outcomes has been scant (Waldfogel, 2000b; McGowen & Walsh, 1998). However, recent federal legislation and new federal monitoring procedures have mandated that child welfare systems measure outcomes and increase their accountability to the general public that supports them and the children and families they serve (U.S. General Accounting Office, 2004).

The literature has called for increased research in effective child welfare practice (Poertner, MacDonald & Murray, 2000; Epstein, 1999). However, it is unclear whether administrators, supervisors and workers are aware of, or use such research findings in their agencies when it is available. Further, the literature has not documented a consistent use of evidence-based practice in child welfare (Usher & Wildfire, 2003). We don't know, for instance, what attitudes child welfare staff have about evidence-based practice, or how it may impact their work with families.

Actually achieving evidence-based practice may be elusive in a system that is just beginning to track outcomes for the families and children it serves (Poertner, McDonald & Murray, 2000). Human service organizations historically have relied on the measurement of inputs to document effectiveness (Humphries & Pease, 1992), or process/outputs, rather than the outcomes currently being called for; and the transformation to outcomes measurement will require purposeful change in organizations (Neuman, 2003; Martin, 2000).

EVIDENCE-BASED PRACTICE IN SOCIAL WORK

Social work has the opportunity to build on years of experience in the medical field's work to establish evidence-based practice. Sackett and colleagues (1997) defined as the "... conscientious, explicit, and judicious use of current best evidence in making decisions about the care of individuals." (p. 2). They identified three hallmarks that are as appropriate for social work as they are for medicine: (1) individual assessment; (2) identify the best available evidence to inform the current, specific client and situation; and (3) consideration of the values and expressed expectation of that client (Sackett et al., 1997) in decisions made and action taken in the professional capacity.

Whether social work is, or should be, moving toward evidence-based practice is debated in the literature. Gambrill (1999, 2001) asserts that social work continues to be an authority-based profession, and practitioners underuse that existing knowledge. She states that we must adopt an evidence-based approach to move forward, while Webb (2001) disputes the notion that practitioners will change their practice, even when made aware of research findings. Others assert social work "evidence" is fallible (Witkin & Harrison, 2001), and have found a lack of consensus on what constitutes it (MacDonald, 1997; Crisp, 2004). Angel (2003) makes the argument that evidence-based practice promotes a reductionist view of people and that the field of child welfare is too complex to benefit from an emphasis on only empirically-proven programs. However, this is based on a very narrow view on what evidence should be considered.

The literature is full of references proclaiming that social work practice is not evidence-based (Cheatham, 1987; Fischer, 1993; Kirk & Penka, 1992; Richey, Blythe & Berlin, 1987; Rosen, 1994; Rosen, Proctor, Morrow-Howell & Staudt, 1995). Shaw and Shaw (1997) studied narrative accounts from social workers on what evidence they used to determine if their practice is expected, and found that emotional rewards, incremental movement in the case, lack of harm inflicted, and confirmation by colleagues were prevalent sources. In a statewide evaluation of seventeen family support programs, Carrilio, Packard and Clapp (2003) found that programs did not consistently use their information systems' data, despite the provision of training and technical assistance to do so. Their proposed solution lies in promoting organizational culture change to one that values information, quality performance and measured results. Others have called for research into methods of promoting critical thinking and research-based decision-making in practice

(Gambrill, 2000; Gibbs & Gambrill, 2002; Howard & Jenson, 1999; MacDonald, 1998; Rosen & Proctor, 2003).

If we believe that outcomes would be improved if child protection workers applied empirical data in their practice, social work would do well to take note of the medical field's example. Technological systems have been built making research-based practice information available to practitioners (Schorr & Auspos, 2003; Cannon & Kilburn, 2003). Barratt (2003) collected data from 100 professional staff on how evidence-based practice can be supported in social agencies, and found that resources to support it are underdeveloped in the organizations studied. She concludes by wondering whether evidence based practice is realistic in services for families and children.

There is support for a broad interpretation of what may encompass evidence-based practice. Some urge us to consider qualitative or mixed method approaches to evidence-gathering, rather than relying solely on quantitative data (Holloway, 2001; Humphries, 2003). Berlin and Marsh (1993) remind us that if practitioners systematically collect and analyze data of various forms, they are involved in empirically-based practice. Another case study of two community-based child welfare agencies documents how they have promoted an approach to evidence-based practice that is based on systematic development and refinement of practice knowledge (Usher & Wildfire, 2003). Frost (2002) urges us strike a balance in which evidence is pursued within the real world and its limitations. As Rosen (2003) argues, good social work practice is responsive to client needs, outcomes-focused, subject to scrutiny, based on empirical knowledge and evaluated.

THE QUALITY IMPROVEMENT CENTERS– THE CHILDREN'S BUREAU'S INITIATIVE FOR EBP

Funding from the U.S. Department of Health and Human Services (DHHS), established the Southern Regional Quality Improvement Center for Child Protection (SR QIC) in 2001 in order to promote innovation, evidence-based practice improvements and to disseminate information on promising practices. The SR QIC is one of four centers nationally which have been funded to test their ability to achieve these outcomes. This is clearly an attempt to increase evidence-based practice in public child welfare. With these factors in mind and within the framework set by the Children's Bureau, the SR QIC established the following objectives, each of which are closely related to the promotion of evidence-based practice:

1. To create regional learning laboratories that will promote collaborative problem-solving, program evaluation, and practice improvement through public agency, university and community partnerships.
2. To promote evidence-based practice, and an outcomes orientation in child welfare delivery systems.
3. To build lasting capacity in the public system by expanding university and community partnerships which yield reinvigorated research and community support for ongoing work, educate future practitioners in state-of-the-art practice, and solidify training partnerships that allow for expanded use of state and federal funding.

A needs assessment was completed to determine which area of child welfare practice would be the focus of the research and demonstration projects. The detail of data collected in this needs assessment has been reported elsewhere (see Collins-Camargo & Groeber, 2003). Based on this data the decision was made to research frontline casework supervision. This is consistent with the findings of a participatory research study examining three groups of social workers to determine what these practitioners saw as barriers to effective practice in child care. Based on their interviews and observations, the authors recommend that agencies must provide models of supervision that promote evidence-based practice (Randall, Cowley & Tomlinson, 2000).

Once the topic of supervision was selected, a survey was conducted by the SR QIC regarding supervision in public child welfare systems in six states (N = 836), and its relationship to effective frontline practice. Based on this survey and the subsequent literature review completed, funded projects ". . . were asked to encompass the following supervisory emphases and activities in the clinical casework supervision models they are testing:

- Scheduled individual or group supervision conferences;
- Promoting enhanced worker critical thinking skills;
- Opportunities for workers to engage in self-reflection, to examine and consider ways to improve their practice;
- Identification of important casework questions that get to the heart of issues related to the family maltreatment and apply the knowledge gained in assessment and treatment;

- Worker skill and focus on evidence-based practice, both in looking to the professional literature for guidance in casework and in the implementation of program evaluation which promote an outcomes orientation to their work with families;
- The establishment of an organizational culture in which support, learning, and clinical supervision and consultation are encouraged; and,
- The use of case review, observation, and similar methods by supervisors to assess worker skill and gauge progress" (Collins-Camargo & Groeber, 2003, p. 24).

Gambrill (1999) emphasized that the skills associated with evidence-based practice include identifying answerable questions, and a process and a source of credible evidence for answering them, critically appraising the evidence obtained, applying the selected evidence to work with clients, and evaluating the outcomes of this intervention. The parallel between these skills, and those emphasized in the SR QIC clinical supervision projects is not accidental. Four projects (in Arkansas, Mississippi, Missouri and Tennessee, and detailed elsewhere in this issue) were funded to test structured, clinical supervision in frontline public child welfare using a public agency/university/community partnership approach. They are focusing on the use of clinical supervision to promote the skills listed above in child welfare workers, along with developing a learning laboratory environment where critical inquiry is promoted, which is another suggested requirement of evidence-based practice (Gambrill, 1999).

SR QIC staff have emphasized the importance of transforming organizational culture in the child welfare agency since the beginning. This culture has been found in the literature to be critical in promoting effective practice, particularly in agencies in which workers may feel vulnerable to external scandal and blaming (Randall, Cowley & Tomlinson, 2000). This could be said to be true of child welfare, as the stakes are very high in this type of practice, and agencies are often blamed by the media when tragedy occurs in families. Hodges and Hernandez (1999) found that the organizational culture is a very important factor in the extent to which client outcome data is valued. In fact, the literature has suggested that changing the culture may be just as important as efforts to develop evidence-based practice skills in individual workers (Crisp, Swerisson & Duckett, 2000), so significant attention has been paid to this feature in our program.

Some of the approaches being tested in the SR QIC projects are specifically grounded in research on techniques for effective promotion of evidence-based practice. Gira and colleagues (2004) review the research on techniques to increase the use of evidence-based information in medicine, and conclude that educational outreach visits, use of local opinion leaders, audit and feedback processes and computer systems showed some effectiveness in changing behavior when monitoring and feedback were present. Multifaceted strategies were most successful. In line with educational outreach visits, two of the SR QIC projects are using a mentoring methodology. All of the projects are using a form of audit and feedback mechanisms, both as a part of their intervention with supervisors and in the clinical supervision techniques being taught. Peer support and consultation networks being built between supervisors may serve a similar purpose to the local opinion leader strategy. Finally two of the projects have used computer-based methods to provide access to information for their participants. If the success of multi-faceted strategies found by Gira and colleagues (2004) holds in our settings, the projects should see at least moderate success in promoting evidence-based practice.

The definition of evidence-based practice promoted in the SR QIC projects is a comprehensive one. As Gambrill (2003) noted, the literature has often offered a very narrow definition such as restricting it to use of empirically validated interventions (e.g., Rosen & Proctor, 2002). The state of empirically validated interventions in child welfare is very limited and at an early stage in development, leading to the need for practitioners to develop a systematic approach to their work in which they are continually evaluating and refining their practice, building on local experiences. This has been piloted in some urban child welfare agencies successfully (Usher & Wildfire, 2003). This approach is consistent with Gambrill's vision–EBP is more than using research findings in practice–it is a process that should integrate evidentiary, ethical, and application in fulfillment of a "systematic, client-oriented vision." (2003, p. 18).

The quasi-experimental research design being employed by the SR QIC for these projects is grounded in a similar notion. It has been noted that much research in child welfare yields inconsistent findings, and a major contributing factor is seen as a poor fit between traditional research models focused on direct causality and the reality of public child welfare which is subject to rampant change and complicated contextual influences (Solomon, 2002). This calls for what Pawson and Tilley (1997) refer to as "realistic"evaluation which is undertaken with the understanding that outcomes are not simply the consequences of an intervention through a traditional causal mechanism, but are also impacted by the interaction between the intervention and "its prevailing contextual condition; i.e., the spatial, geographical or institutional location into which programs are embedded as well as the norms, values and interrelationships which may influence the efficacy of the program" (p. 26).

The projects funded through the SR QIC are engaged in a cross-site evaluation process using pre-established outcomes related to organizational culture, worker and supervisor practice as well as five case outcomes using data from the child welfare agencies information system. Please see Collins-Camargo and Groeber (2004) for detail on the overall cross-site research. Some of the common instrumentation being used in all sites, is particularly relevant to promoting evidence-based practice. The *Self-Efficacy Assessment-Social Work* measures worker self-efficacy in child welfare tasks (Ellett, Ellett & Rugatt, 2003). Its use in the study not only provides data that can be compared across sites, but provides child welfare workers and supervisors with information regarding worker's beliefs about their practice, setting an important expectation of the importance of self-reflection regarding one's skills and their application with clients. Only preliminary findings are available based on analysis of data from this aspect of the research design so it would be premature to report it at this time.

In addition, the SR QIC has conducted focus groups with supervisors in the intervention groups in all sites, part of which is focused on the application of evidence-based practice in the field as a result of the projects. The questions being asked in these focus groups center on outcomes being observed by the supervisors in their practice, that of their workers, and in their clients that they attribute to the intervention. This, too, models the importance of an outcomes-based orientation in child welfare for the participating supervisors.

If We Agree Evidence-Based Practice Is a Good Idea, Why Is It So Difficult to Achieve?

Public agency staff and social work faculty on each of the implementation teams for the four projects have clearly agreed that moving toward evidence-based practice through the use of clinical supervision on the frontline is an important priority. However, numerous challenges have been experienced by SR QIC staff in their attempts to facilitate this process and provide needed technical assistance in the implementation and evaluation of the projects. During the summer of 2004, this author and two colleagues conducted the aforementioned focus groups with each state's intervention group. Seven focus groups were conducted, involving 80 total participants. These focus groups collected data regarding outcomes being observed associated with the clinical supervision projects, and overall, the findings were very encouraging. It is not possible to discuss all of the findings from these focus groups here, but some of the information is relevant to the current topic. One of the questions asked participants for examples of how evidence-based practice was occurring on their work unit. The challenges described below came out of analysis of transcripts from the focus groups, and were supported through the experience of administering these research and demonstration grants. What follows is a brief discussion of each. These challenges may, in fact, represent challenges to the embodiment of evidence-based practice itself in public child welfare.

Lack of Easily Accessible Evidence for Use in Child Welfare Today

Despite the long history of social work practice in child welfare settings, the field has produced a relatively small body of research-based evidence regarding effective interventions (McGowen & Walsh, 1998). Some of this may be related to a characteristic of all social work practice, which is certainly relevant in child welfare: one cannot remove the importance of individual judgment in assessment and decision-making, which is difficult to incorporate into many evidence-based practice approaches (Taylor & White, 2001; Webb, 2001). As Humphries (2003) noted, social work is a moral, social and political activity, which impacts how evidence-based practice can be realized in our field, calling for the use of many types of knowledge. Certainly this is true of child protection. Focus group participants in each state reported that their agency did not provide outcome-focused data from their information system, either at all or in a format enabling them to use it to improve practice on their unit. For example, one participant stated: "That's a shame, because the data is there. I know it's there. It's just not accessible. I've seen it, not [on the worker/unit level] but from the state, and collectively it's there." Some feel unprepared to use the data in a proactive way: "But some of the problem is with the reports we do get, I've had them brought to me through the years–I have no clue what I'm supposed to be doing with them."

Complicating the small but growing body of research evidence in child welfare, is the extent to which child welfare staff may be limited in their ability to access what is out there. One of the partially successful strategies for promoting evidence-based practice in medicine was the use of computer technologies (Gira, Kessler & Poertner, 2004). In our experience, however, some state child welfare staff are not able to use internet-based technologies in their work as the decision to restrict this has been made from their agencies. Some do not even have access to email. Compounding potential lack of adequate hardware or Internet access is the fact that child welfare staff may not have time to peruse the professional journals to stay current on research findings impacting their work. The crisis-driven nature of their work certainly impacts this.

Do Child Welfare Agencies Really Want Inquiring Minds on Their Frontline?

During the focus groups, a recurring theme in all states was reference to barriers originating in the central administration in the agency. Participants from each noted what they described as a punitive approach with the field, which may well be an impediment to an organizational culture promoting learning and an outcomes-orientation. In some states, supervisors felt their agencies remained overly reliant on reporting systems that focused more on process rather than outcomes. Some questioned whether the agencies were really committed to positive change. One participant summarized it this way: "We get the vision–we know that there is a vision. We're the forerunners of the vision, so we know that there is a vision for the agency, and we want [the administration] to know that we are positive. It's not them against us." This is consistent with findings reported by Carrilio, Packard and Clapp (2003) in that middle and upper management opposition can be a significant barrier to evidence-based practice. In large public agencies, a change in administrative philosophy may be needed to move away from top down decision-making and into a milieu where questioning from the bottom up is encouraged.

INSTITUTIONAL REVIEW BOARDS' DISCOMFORT WITH APPLIED RESEARCH IN PUBLIC AGENCIES

Part of the overall intent of the SR QIC learning laboratory model is to promote a comfort level with evaluation methodology and research in the public agency. Two of the involved university institutional review boards (IRBs), however, presented significant barriers to moving forward with our research. Although IRB approval was eventually obtained in all sites, a central theme was convincing them that there would not be employment-related risks experienced by supervisors in the intervention group, and that these participants really could provide meaningful informed consent despite the fact that they were employees of a public agency. Human subjects protections are certainly critical to our work and should not be under-emphasized. However, we must be able to perform research in public bureaucracies, and to do so we cannot hold such studies to the level of protections offered in laboratory settings. The nature of public child welfare agencies require that we work to educate IRBs in terms of what is possible, and to use creative approaches to minimizing risk, if we are to substantially increase the volume of research being conducted in these agencies, and, in turn, the body of evidence available to practitioners.

Difficulty Maintaining and Measuring Treatment Fidelity in Large Public Agencies

While not noted in the focus group data, a theme noted in process evaluation data collected by SR QIC staff relates to treatment fidelity on several levels. Project staff reported finding it difficult to measure fidelity to the practice model being tested. Supervisors certainly noted in each of the focus groups their inability to implement all aspects of the clinical supervision model they had been taught. Projects have taken pains to limit additional data collection from already overloaded child welfare workers and supervisors. At the same time, project and SR QIC staff have repeatedly had to de-rail attempts by the agencies to prematurely roll out project interventions statewide, to avoid contamination of the research. In a field where administrators are hungry for strategies to improve services–and widespread change is afoot–they may be desperate for innovative approaches with good potential. Organizational culture change may be necessary to create an environment in which research can be conducted and data gathered for an adequate amount of time before replication begins, so that we can have a better sense of whether the evidence supports them.

Revolving Door of Public Agency Administrators

The political nature of the work in public agencies brings with it frequent changes in leadership. Process evaluation data collected through key informant interviews by the SR QIC indicates that all four projects have experienced an on-going problem with this. They find themselves educating new administrators on what we are trying to achieve, and the merits of the research design on a regular basis. This revolving door of leadership may prove a problem for obtaining commitment to the organizational changes necessary to promote evidence-based practice in the field of child welfare.

THE CHASM BETWEEN RESEARCH AND PRACTICE LIVES ON

Gray (2001) noted that an important lesson social work can learn from medicine is the importance of bridging the chasm between research and practice. The philosophical approach adopted by the SR QIC requiring a partnership between the public agency and the university for each funded project was designed to begin to force this issue. Process-related data shows that this continues to be a problem. Collaboration challenges required the highest percentage of technical assistance contacts with grantees during implementation year two (22%). This was a more significant need than research/evaluation, implementation, fiscal, reporting or communication issues. In addition, key informant interviews conducted as part of process evaluation noted that this represented an ongoing challenge.

The agencies' openness to partnership with university social work programs, and perhaps by extension to the research community, may be complicated by the fact that the public child welfare agencies in most of these states do not require a social work educational background in their staff. In addition, SR QIC staff have observed a trend in at least half of the universities to see these projects as "training" initiatives rather than research endeavors, and have thereby devalued the effort. It is unclear the extent to which this may be exacerbated by a negative attitude among some faculty regarding child welfare research in general, or whether it is specific to this program. Regardless, many factors potentially impact this division between research and practice in our field.

What Does "Evidence-Based Practice" Really Mean?

The lack of clarity noted in the literature regarding a definition of evidence-based practice (e.g., Crisp, 2004; MacDonald, 1997) was echoed in the focus groups conducted by the SR QIC. Gambrill (2003) cited Dawson and Berry (2002) and Corcoran (2000) as examples of articles on the topic not clearly defining the notion. Without exception, supervisors participating in the SR QIC focus group had difficulty understanding the term "evidence-based practice" and applying it to work in their field. They had to be prompted by repeated explanation of the definition to generate examples noted later in this paper. One participant stated "Evidence based decision making is good, and that's what we need to be doing, but I haven't been able to apply it." In one state, the participants of both focus groups were unable to discuss it at all in a meaningful way. This is clearly an area in which our projects can stand to improve.

From the point of view of the SR QIC projects, evidence-based practice includes not just the narrow application of research-based findings in practice, but also, having an outcomes-based orientation in one's work with clients, employing single system designs or other methods of determining that the worker's intervention is making a difference on an individual case level; self-reflection; effectively using ethical decision-making; using agency data systems to inform practice; and, using personal, case and organizational goal-setting and on-going monitoring of incremental progress. Before practitioners can actually perform evidence-based practice they need to (1) understand what it means in the context of the agency in question; (2) believe that it is an important aspect of best and ethical practice; (3) believe that it is valued in the organization or work unit and that the environment will allow and support it; and, (4) possess expectancy valance, believing that performing in this manner will have the likelihood of positive impact on families.

EVOLVING SOLUTIONS TO ANSWER CHALLENGES

Despite these challenges, data on regarding evidence-based practice from focus groups demonstrated that it is happening on some level. Participants from three of the four states were able to provide examples of staff demonstrating an appreciation of an analytic approach to their practice. This was truly a central theme from the data gathered: "I think the analyzing focus has been a big change, at least for me personally. Analyzing what I'm doing, analyzing what the workers are doing. ...What's working, what's not working ... I think the analyzing [of] the work at all levels, has improved." In addition, participants from individual states provided examples in the following categories: seeking client feedback; a positive attitude regarding peer review; supervisors gathering data on what workers need; tracking evidence of behavioral change in clients. For example, participants stated: "On-going workers have more chance to be self-reflective on whether the family is improving and meeting goals–constantly reviewing. We have to teach some of that"; "It's hanging in there, and trying to find strategies that work. It's the workers thinking outside the box and . . . they are all committed, and it has a good chance of working now." After only one year of implementation, this is encouraging.

Reflecting on the progress we have made within the SR QIC, it seems important that evidence-based practice be seen as a process–an approach. As suggested by Haynes, Devereaux and Guyalt, it is ". . . a guide for thinking about how decisions should be made." (2002, p. 2). In this context, two strategies seem important. First, in child welfare agencies the Child and Family Services Review process provides an important impetus for adoption of such an approach. The federally motivated emphasis on outcomes can be an important stimulant of organizational change.

Secondly, our projects would seem to be in a good place to promoted evidence-based practice, as they target frontline supervision. Understanding the tremendous need for organizational learning in their staff (in effect, evidence-based practice), according to Cohen and Austin (1994) child welfare agencies must strengthen four capabilities: diagnosis/problem definition and questioning practice realities; invention or challenging the status quo; the ability to test ideas in practice; and generalization. The potential influence of supervisors on this development is clear. Bernard and Goodyear (2004) assert that supervision has two purposes: "to foster the supervisee's professional development . . . [and] to ensure client welfare" (p. 12). This could be interpreted that to ensure client welfare requires evidence-based practice, so the conceptual connection between these two seems sound. Evidence-based practice flows from the facilitation of an organizational culture that promotes it, and the direct influence supervisors can have on the development of worker skills in this area is clear.

Without question, our emphasis on organizational culture change to one focused on learning has been important to our success. Our research and demonstration projects were designed by the Children's Bureau to encourage evidence-based practice–researching interventions in the child welfare agency before formally replicating them. SR QIC staff provided structure to the projects intended to enable them to adhere fairly consistently to the research design, and project staff have responded well to this. It has been noted in the literature that organizational culture and structure are required for evidence-based practice to occur in frontline social work (Blumenfield & Epstein, 2001; Rapp & Poertner, 1992).

The parallel process between the SR QIC-project, project-supervisor, and supervisor-frontline worker levels is not accidental. We have attempted to create a learning laboratory atmosphere amongst the projects so that they could mirror it in their state and within their intervention. The findings of our summative evaluation are yet to be determined. However, these lessons learned during the journey of administering projects aimed at promoting evidence-based practice may have application today to others venturing in this direction. Certainly the child welfare field must move forward in adopting practical yet forward-thinking approaches to evidence-based practice. The complex and public nature of this area of social work practice, and the lives of our most vulnerable, who depend on it, require creative and diligent solutions. Our focus group participants may have captured the spirit of this better than this author can:

- "It's all about learning, improving, getting better, growing, striving to a higher level of performance."–an Arkansas supervisor
- "I want to be the best supervisor I can be, but I'm not, and one thing that I believe this project has helped me to learn is that this is ongoing."–a Mississippi supervisor
- "I think we are being forced to examine ourselves as an entity as a whole and as individuals. I think it is going to provide the best opportunity for growth in the agency because we if we're honest with ourselves it will be easier to be honest with the workers and everybody else that we work with and I think it will create better outcomes."–a Missouri supervisor
- "I think a lot of things we take for granted, and we really need to be looking at what we know. We need to be looking past, and really thinking about what we're doing."–a Tennessee supervisor

REFERENCES

Angel, B. O. (2003). Evidence-based programs: Forms of knowledge and outlooks on people in social work. *Nordisk Sosialt Arbeid, 23*(2), 66-72.

Barratt, M. (2003). Organizational support for evidence-based practice within child and family social work: A collaborative study. *Child & Family Social Work, 8*(2), 143-151.

Berlin, S.G., & Marsh, J.C. (1993). *Informing practice decisions*. New York: Macmillan.

Bernard, J. M., & Goodyear, R. K. (2004). *Fundamentals of clinical supervision*, 3rd edition. Boston, MA: Pearson Education, Inc.

Blumenfield, S., & Epstein, I. (2001). Introduction: Promoting and maintaining a reflective professional staff in a hospital-based social work department. *Social Work in Health Care, 33*(3-4), 1-13.

Cannon, J. S., & Kilburn, M. R. (2003). Meeting decision-makers' needs for evidence-based information on child and family policy. *Journal of Policy Analysis and Management, 22(*4), 665-669.

Carrilio, T. E.; Packard, T., & Clapp, J.D. (2003). Nothing in–nothing out: Barriers to the use of performance data in social service programs. *Administration in Social Work, 27*(4), 61-76.

Cheatham, J.M. (1987). The empirical evaluation of clinical practice: a survey of our groups of practitioners. *Journal of Social Service Research, 10*, 163-177.

Collins-Camargo, C., & Groeber, C. (2003). Adventures in Partnership: Using Learning Laboratories to Enhance Frontline Supervision in Child Welfare. *Professional Development: The International Journal of Continuing Social Work Education, 6*(1 & 2), 17-31.

Corcoran, J. (2000). *Evidence-based social work practice with families: A life-span approach*. New York: Springer.

Crisp, B.R. (2004). Evidence-based practice and the boarders of data in the global information era. *Journal of Social Work Education, 40*(1), 73-86.

Crisp, B.R., Swerissen, H., & Duckette, S.J. (2000). Four approaches to capacity building in health: Consequences for measurement and accountability. *Health Promotion International, 15*, 99-107.

Dawson, K., & Berry, M. (2002). Engaging families in child welfare services: An evidence-based approach to best practice. *Child Welfare, 81*(2), 293-317.

Ellett, A., Ellett, C., & Rugutt, J. (2003). *A study of personal and organizational factors contributing to employee retention and turnover in child welfare in Georgia: Final project report.* Unpublished manuscript. University of Georgia.

Epstein, W. (1999). *Children who could have been: The Legacy of child welfare in wealthy America.* Madison, WI: University of Wisconsin Press.

Fischer, J. (1993). Empirically-based practice: The end of ideology? *Journal of Social Service Research, 18*, 19-64.

Frost, N. (2002). A problematic relationship? Evidence and practice in the workplace. *Social Work & Social Sciences Review, 10*(1), 38-50.

Gambrill, E. (1999). Evidence-based practice: an alternative to authority-based practice. *Families in Society: The Journal of Contemporary Human Services, 80*(4), 341-350.

Gambrill, E. (2000). Therole of critical thinking in evidence-based social work. In P. Allen-Meares & C. Garvin, (Eds.), *The handbook of social work direct practice* (pp. 43-63). Thousand Oaks, CA: Sage Publications.

Gambrill, E. (2001). Social work: An authority-based profession. *Research on Social Work Practice, 11*(2), 166-176.

Gambrill, E. (2003). From the editor:; Evidence-based practice: Sea change or the emperor's new clothes? *Journal of Social Work Education, 39*(1), 3-23.

Gibbs, L., & Gambrill, E. (2002). Evidence-based practice: Counterarguments to objections. *Research on Social Work Practice, 12*(3), 452-477.

Gira, E. C., Kessler, M., & Poertner, J. (2004). Influencing social workers to use research evidence in practice: Lessons from medicine and the allied health professions. *Research on Social Work Practice, 14*(2), 68-80.

Gray, J. A. M. (2001). The origin of evidence-based practice. In A. Edwards & G. Elwyn (Eds.), *Evidence-informed client choice* (pp. 19-33). New York: Oxford University Press.

Haynes, R. B., Devereaux, P.J., & Guyatt, G. H. (2002). Clinical expertise in the era of evidence-based medicine and patient choice. [Editorial]. *ACP Journal Club,* March/April, *136*, 1-7.

Hodges, S., & Hernandez, M. (1999). How organizational culture influences outcome information utilization. *Evaluation and Program Planning, 22*, 183-197.

Hollway, W. (2001). The psycho-social subject in "evidence-based practice." *Journal of Social Work Practice, 15*(1), 9-23.

Howard, M. O., & Jenson, J. M. (1999). Clinical practice guidelines: Should social work develop them? *Research on Social Work Practice, 9*, 234-259.

Humphries, B. (2003). What else counts as evidence in evidence-based social work? *Social Work Education, 22*(1), 81-91.

Humphries, C., & Pease, K. (1992). Effectiveness measurement in the probation service: A view from the troops. *Howard Journal, 13*(2), 31-52.

Kirk, S.A., & Penka, C.E. (1992). Research utilization and MSW education: A decade of progress? In A. J. Grasso & I. Epstein (Eds.), *Research utilization in the social services* (pp. 407-421). Binghamton, NY: Haworth Press.

MacDonald, G. (1998). Promoting evidence-based practice in child protection. *Clinical Child Psychology and Psychiatry, 3*(1), 71-85.

Martin, L. L. (2000). Budgetng for outcomes in state human agencies. *Administration in Social Work, 24*(3), 71-88.

McGowen, B., & Walsh, E., (2000). Policy changes for child welfare in the new century. *Child Welfare,. 79*(1), 11-28.

Moore, T. D., Rapp, C.A., & Roberts, B (2000). Improving child welfare performance through supervisory use of client outcome data. *Child Welfare, 79*(5), 475-497.

Munro, E. (1999). Common errors of reasoning in child protection work. *Child Abuse and Neglect, 23*(8), 745-758.

Neuman, K. M. (2003). Developing a comprehensive outcomes management program: A ten step process. *Administration in Social Work, 27*(1), 5-21.

Patti, R. (1987). Managing for service effectiveness in social welfare: Towards a performance model. *Administration in Social Work, 11*, 7-22.

Pawson, R., & Tilley, N. (1997). *Realistic evaluation*. Thousand Oaks: Sage Publications.

Poertner, J., McDonald, T., & Murray, C. (2000). Child welfare outcomes revisited. *Children and Youth Services Review, 22*(9/10), 789-810.

Randall, J., Cowley, P., & Tomlinson, P. (2000). Overcoming barriers to effective practice in child care. *Child and Family Social Work, 5*, 343-352.

Rapp, C., & Poertner, J. (1992). *Social administration: A client centered approach*. New York: Longman Publishing.

Richey, C. A., Blythe, B. J., & Berlin, S. B. (1987). Do social workers evaluate their practice? *Social Work Research & Abstracts, 23*(2), 14-20.

Rosen, A. (2003). Evidence-based social work practice: Challenges and promise. *Social Work Research, 27*(4), 197-208.

Rosen, A. (1994). Knowledge use in direct practice. *Social Service Review, 68*, 561-577.

Rosen, A., & Proctor, E.K. (Eds). (2003). *Developing practice guidelines for social work intervention: Issues, methods, and research agenda*. New York: Columbia University Press.

Rosen, A., Proctor, E.K., Morrow-Howell, N., & Staudt, M. (1995). Rationales for practice decisions: Variations in knowledge used by decision task and social work service. *Research on Social Work Practice, 5*, 501-523.

Rossi, P., Schuerman, J., & Budde, S. (1999). Understanding decisions about child maltreatment. *Evaluation Review. 23*(6), 579-598.

Sackett, D.L., Richardson, W.S., Rosenberg, W., & Haynes, R. B. (1997). *Evidence-based medicine: How to practice and teach EMB.* New York: Churchill Livingstone.

Schorr, L. B., & Auspos, P. (2003). Usable information about what works: Building a broader and deeper knowledge base. *Journal of Policy Analysis and Management, 22*(4), 669-676.

Shaw, I., & Shaw, A. (1997). Game plans, busses, and sheer luck: Doing well in social work. *Social Work Research, 21*(2), 69-80.

Solomon, B. (2002). Accountability in public child welfare: Linking program theory, program specification and program evaluation. *Children and Youth Services Review, 24*(6/7), 385-407.

Taylor, C., & White, S. (2001). Knowledge, truth and reflexivity: The problem of judgment in social work. *Journal of Social Work, 1*(1), 37-59.

United States General Accounting Office (2004). *Child And Family Service Reviews: Better Use of Data and Improved Guidance Could Enhance HHS's Oversight of State Performance* (Report No. GAO04-333). Washington, DC: United States General Accounting Office.

Usher, C. L., & Wildfire, J.B. (2003). Evidence-based practice in community-based child welfare systems. *Child Welfare, 82*(5), 597-614.

Waldfogel, J. (1998). Rethinking the paradigm for child protection. *Future of Children, 8*(1), 104-119.

Waldfogel, J. (2000a). Reforming Child Protective Services. *Child Welfare, 79*(1), 43-58.

Waldfogel, J. (2000b). Child welfare research: How adequate are the data? *Children and Youth Services Review, 22*(9/10), 705-741.

Webb, S. A. (2001). Some considerations on the validity of evidence-based practice in social work. *British Journal of Social Work, 31*, 57-79.

Webb, S. (2002). Evidence-based practice and decision analysis in social work: An implementation model. *Journal of Social Work, 2*(1), 45-63.

Webster, D., Needell, B., & Wildfire, J. (2002). Data are your friends: foster child welfare agency self0evalution in Los Angeles County with the Family to Family Initiative. *Children and Youth Services Review, 24*, 471-484.

Witkin, S.L., & Harrison, W.D. (2001). Whose evidence and for what purpose? [Editorial]. *Social Work, 46*, 293-296.

doi:10.1300/J394v04n03_03

Linking Self-Efficacy Beliefs to Employee Retention in Child Welfare: Implications for Practice, Theory, and Research

Alberta J. Ellett, PhD

SUMMARY. This article describes the results of a two-state study of relationships between child welfare employees' intentions to remain employed in child welfare and their self-efficacy beliefs about their capabilities to accomplish core work tasks. Linkages between self-efficacy motivation and persistence and intent to remain employed in child welfare were also examined. The development of the study measures and the results of data analyses pertaining to their empirical structures and scale reliabilities for a large sample (n = 941) of child welfare staff are described. Major findings of the study confirmed the hypothesized, positive relationships between child welfare employees' self-efficacy beliefs and their intentions to remain employed in child welfare. These findings replicated across the two states. Implications of the findings for practice, theory development, and future research in child welfare are discussed.
doi:10.1300/J394v04n03_04

Alberta J. Ellett is affiliated with the School of Social Work, Tucker Hall, University of Georgia, Athens, GA 30602 (E-mail: aellett@uga.edu).

[Haworth co-indexing entry note]: "Linking Self-Efficacy Beliefs to Employee Retention in Child Welfare: Implications for Practice, Theory, and Research." Ellett, Alberta J. Co-published simultaneously in the *Journal of Evidence-Based Social Work* (The Haworth Press, Inc.) Vol. 4, No. 3/4, 2007, pp. 39-68; and: *Developing an Empirically Based Practice Inititative: A Case Study in CPS Supervision* (ed: Jenny L. Jones, and Paul Sundet) The Haworth Press, 2007, pp. 39-68. Single or multiple copies of this article are available for a fee from The Haworth Document Delivery Service [1-800-HAWORTH, 9:00 a.m. - 5:00 p.m. (EST). E-mail address: docdelivery@haworthpress.com].

Available online at http://jebsw.haworthpress.com

doi:10.1300/J394v04n03_04

KEYWORDS. Self-efficacy, child welfare, child protection, employee retention, supervision

INTRODUCTION

The practice of social work, and child welfare in particular, are difficult work contexts to effect child safety, permanence and well being with perhaps the nation's most needy and troubled families and youth (Ellett & Ellett, 1997; Hopkins, Mudrick, & Rudolph, 1999; Rycus & Hughes, 1994). Public child welfare is unique among social work areas of practice in that the vast majority of clients are involuntary and interventions primarily take place in clients' homes. Child welfare clients often live in low income neighborhoods and areas in which problems are often dealt with in violent ways, adding additional stress to an already complex job for workers to attend to not only child safety, but to their own personal safety as well. Well-intentioned child welfare staff are often the target of public, judicial, media and government criticism in serious and child fatality cases. This criticism is made without the understanding that child welfare staff are working to carry out federal and state mandates in a system that is under funded, under staffed and most agencies have established inadequate credentials for personnel to carry out this vital work. There are limited promotional opportunities for child welfare staff essentially leading them to *dead-end* jobs rather than a career or profession (Ellett & Ellett; Hopkins et al.; Ellett & Leighninger, in press; Louisiana Work Group, 2000; Rycus & Hughes, 1994; U.S. Government Accounting Office, 1995). Given this work context, annual turnover among child welfare employees is 20-40% nationally, and as high as 100% in some counties [American Public Human Services Association (APHSA), 2001, 2005; U.S. General Accounting Office (GAO), 2003].

Over the past three decades, burnout and job stress have been the primary focus of the literature that attempts to explain turnover of child welfare employees (Aber, 1983; Anderson, 2000; Dickinson & Perry, 2002; Drake & Yadama, 1996; Fryer, Miyoshi, & Thomas, 1989; Harrison, 1995; Jayaratne & Chess, 1984a,b; 1986; Kern, McFadden, Baumann, 1993; Lewandowski, 2003; Liederman, 1998; McMahon, 1999; Mor Barak, Nissly, & Levin, 2001; Samantrai, 1992; Scully, 1983; Tett & Meyer, 1993). Focusing on employees who have left public child welfare is somewhat problematic because these employees may be some of the most dysfunctional members of child welfare organizations. An additional problem is that published studies of employee burnout and turnover seldom conceptually define what burnout is, and results of these studies have been rather inconclusive in attributing employee turnover to burnout. Indeed, Söderfeldt, Söderfeldt, and Warg (1995) speculate that burnout may be a socially acceptable way to give up on a job.

STUDYING EMPLOYEE RETENTION

While burnout has received considerable attention in the literature, far less attention has been given to studies designed to better understand the *holding power* of social work organizations, and personal and organizational factors related to employees' *intentions to remain employed in child welfare,* studies which may yield more useful information for child welfare organizations (Cicero-Reese & Black, 1997; Dickinson & Perry; 2002; Helfgott, 1991; Ellett, 2000; Jayaratne & Chess, 1984a; Reagh, 1994; Rycraft, 1994; Vinokur-Kaplan, 1991). Studying factors related to employee retention may generate important information having implications for pre-service education, employee selection, supervision and support, and strengthening organizational culture. For example, in a small qualitative exploratory study of 23 child welfare caseworkers whose average length of employment was 11 years, Rycraft (1994) identified four factors influencing retention. These were (a) goodness of fit of worker skills, interests, and the specific job responsibilities with professional knowledge, skill and ability; (b) mission, i.e., caseworker commitment to helping others especially abused/neglected children and their families, and overcoming barriers to provide intervention; (c) supportive supervision appropriate to worker skill level and experience; and (d) personal and professional investments in public child welfare, and the investments of agency in them.

Through written life histories, results of the Maslach Burnout Inventory, and interviews of 18 public child welfare workers, Reagh (1994) found that child welfare workers who remain in child welfare typically: (a) were altruistic, (b) were personally identified with public child welfare; (c) had a desire to make a difference; (d) found meaning in their work; (e) felt a strong sense of accomplishment; (f) saw themselves as constantly growing and learning; (g) received support from their colleagues; and (h) had a strong need to feel valued, rewarded, and appreciated. Reagh also identified a very fine line between staying and leaving and these characteristics. That is, all workers in the study had experienced burnout at some level. Staying and leaving work in child welfare were not viewed as opposites, but were viewed as decisions that were only different depending upon the way the individual processes work experiences. The workers interviewed in the Reagh study also recommended that mature workers could effectively serve as mentors for new staff to improve retention rates.

To document the importance of mentoring to employee retention, Collins (1994) conducted a survey among 631 social workers who provided internship supervision of MSW students in 300 human services settings. She was interested in examining whether mentorship had a similar positive impact on career development as had been shown to be the case in business and education settings, and in the organizational and developmental psychology literatures. Her results showed that both the mentor and protégée roles in mentoring settings had a significant impact on career success, career satisfaction and income levels for the mentor and protégée, when these individuals were compared to those who had not participated in a mentorship.

In summarizing the literature reviewed related to retention in public child welfare, only a few, small qualitative studies had been attempted to empirically identify or discuss factors related to retention (Reagh, 1994; Rycraft, 1994) prior to 2000 and much of the retention literature was in the form of recommendations, was speculative, and/or included only small scale research studies. More recently, studies of Title IV-E graduates' retention have begun to appear in the literature (Brown, Chavkin, & Peterson, 2002; Cicero-Reese & Black, 1997; Dickinson & Perry, 2002; Gansle & Ellett, 2002; Hopkins et al., 1999, Jones, 2002; Lewandowsk, 1998; Robin & Hollister, 2002). The literature reflects a variety of recommendations about improving retention in child welfare, but few actual research studies, and no large-scale quantitative or qualitative studies prior to 2000. Thus, a lot of professional advice and suggestions about ways in which retention might be enhanced and turnover prevented is available. However, few studies to provide an empirical basis for this advice have been completed.

The retention literature identifies mentoring, organizational support, reduced caseloads and other structures framing practice as important to strengthen employee retention in child welfare. However, this literature offers no deep or theory-based explanations as to how and why these structures influence the behavior of child welfare staff, their on-the-job experiences, and ultimately their decisions to remain employed in this difficult and challenging work context. One personal characteristic that has received rather wide research support as a strong factor influencing human behavior in a variety of contexts is self-efficacy (Bandura, 1997). This important characteristic mediating linkages between human behavior and the environment is described in the section that follows.

SELF-EFFICACY

There is a long and rich history in the psychology literature of concern for human self-regulation which "is the capacity of people to think about their future, set goals, develop plans to attain these goals, and regulate their own behavior based on these goals and plans" (Maddux, 1999, p. 17). Theories of self-regulation have at their core various conceptions of the extent to which the individual expects that specific behaviors will produce specific outcomes and accomplish personal goals, and the role that valuing outcomes plays in developing expectancies. Within the larger domain of expectancy theory and the literature of social-cognitive psychology, an important theoretical construct that has received a considerable amount of attention during the past three decades is self-efficacy. A pioneer in self-efficacy theory development and research is the social-cognitive psychologist, Albert Bandura. In discussing the important role that human self-efficacy plays in determining behavior in a wide variety of settings, Bandura (1997) states:

> *perceived self-efficacy refers to beliefs in one's capabilities to organize and execute courses of action to produce given attainments* . . . (and self-efficacy beliefs) . . . influence the courses of action people choose to pursue, how much effort they put forth in given endeavors, how long they will persist in the face of obstacles and failure, their resilience to adversity, whether their thought patterns are self-hindering or self-aiding, how much stress and depression they experience in coping with taxing environmental demands, and the level of accomplishments they realize. (p. 3)

Bandura concludes that people are more strongly influenced by their personal beliefs than objective facts, which impacts their level of motivation, feelings, and behavior. People desire and often expend great effort to gain control over their life circumstances. It is their belief that particular actions cause expected results that motivates much of their behavior. Clearly, within the context of the difficulties surrounding work in child welfare, strengthening the self-efficacy beliefs of professional staff becomes an important concern.

Bandura (1997) makes the argument that persons can exercise considerable influence and control over their own behavior and choices of action. Thus, an individual may believe a particular behavior will produce a given outcome. But if the individual has weak self-efficacy beliefs about capabilities to execute the behavior, the behavior will not occur and the outcome will not be achieved. Similarly, if an individual believes that an outcome can be attained (outcome expectancy) and that the individual possesses the capabilities to accomplish the task (efficacy expectations), the individual will persevere even in the face of repeated failures.

Acquired knowledge and skill are essential in the development of personal beliefs that performing particular actions will lead to expected outcomes. Self-efficacy theory predicts that without necessary cognitive and behavioral skills (competence, professional knowledge and practice skills in the case of social work), no amount of self-efficacy will lead to task accomplishment (Bandura, 1997). People approach and engage in tasks or activities for which they believe they possess the capability to perform successfully and avoid those for which they do not believe they have the capability to succeed.

Bandura (1997) depicts the theory of self-efficacy as a complex process of self-persuasion, which links knowledge acquisition, personal beliefs about capabilities, and subsequent behavior. Efficacy beliefs emanate from four primary sources: (a) enactive mastery experiences (success or failure at tasks), (b) vicarious learning experiences (watching others who are successful or unsuccessful in performing tasks), (c) verbal persuasion (from others or self), and (d) physiological/affective states (which may be pleasant or unpleasant). Thus, human agency and the self-efficacy belief system is developed through the dynamic, reciprocal interplay among personal beliefs (possessing cognitive and affective elements), the environment, and subsequent behavior, a dynamic system Bandura has termed *triadic reciprocal causation.*

Generality vs. Specificity of Self-Efficacy

Early studies of self-efficacy held that the construct was situational and task specific and could not be generalized across situations and tasks like self concept, self-esteem, locus of control, and other self systems. More recently, the literature addresses self-efficacy beliefs as part of a system of cognitively structured experiences and reflective thought. This view conceptualizes self-efficacy as consisting of more generalized rather than highly specific beliefs (Bandura, 1997; Bandura, Adams, & Beyer, 1977; Johnson, 1999; Zimmerman, 1989). Self-efficacy beliefs are also considered to vary in levels (task difficulty), strength (effort and persistence), and generality (across situations and tasks). Thus, across different domains in which individuals function, there is no exact, predictable relationship between efficacy beliefs, expectations related to performance outcomes (what accrues to the individual), and subsequent behavior. Self-efficacy develops as a dynamic, generative process and mastery experience relative to performance and accomplishing outcomes can lead to the development of more generalized self-efficacy in a performance domain. Thus, strong self-efficacy beliefs about accomplishing child welfare domain outcomes build upon success in many areas of practice (in child protective, foster care, adoption services).

In Bandura's (1997) view, it is the affective and evaluative states that follow actions performed that represent outcomes that accrue to the individual. These outcomes can be either positive and reinforce and reward the individual, or negative and discourage the individual. It is these outcomes that the individual subsequently strives for, rather than particular behaviors or performance targets. Most outcome research generally measures or evaluates actions, tasks or the product of actions and tasks. The strength of perceived self-efficacy according to Bandura is important to the individual's level of effort, persistence in overcoming obstacles, resilience to continue when unsuccessful, and accomplishments. People develop personal standards through which they regulate their own behavior and participate in things from which they derive the greatest satisfaction and sense of self-reward and fulfillment. Thus, as an individual's specific areas of child welfare practice occur, skills, and abilities are reinforaced, and self-efficiacy across practice domains is strengthened.

Self-Efficacy and Social Work

The personal construct of self-efficacy fits social work's study of the person in the environment, and expands it to include reciprocity between personal characteristics, the environment and behavior. Thus, self-efficacy is not a fixed character or trait, but varies considerably within different areas of functioning and within different contexts. For example, a child welfare employee with the requisite knowledge and skills may have strong beliefs in their capabilities to accurately assess parenting ability and weak self-efficacy to work with judges and the courts. Self-efficacy is generative, dynamic, and contextually bound (Bandura, 1997).

According to self-efficacy research, individuals approach situations about which they feel competent and confident and avoid those about which they do not. This phenomenon may explain why social work students with child welfare stipends who were able to find employment in child welfare agencies studied by Vinokur-Kaplin (1987 & 1991), reported high levels of satisfaction in their jobs. The stronger are an individual's self-efficacy beliefs, the greater their efforts, persistence, and resilience to overcome obstacles and barriers (Bandura, 1997; Pajares, 1996).

Studies of self-efficacy were just beginning to appear in the social work literature at the time of the 2000 study reported in this article. Holden (1991) may have published the first article on self-efficacy within social work using a meta-analysis of health related outcomes in 56 studies. There appears to be a 5-year gap in the appearance of self-efficacy studies in the social work literature between 1991 and 1996 when Holden, Cuzzi, Rutter, Rosenberg and Chernack (1996) and Cuzzi, Holden, Rutter, Rosenberg, and Chernack (1996) published the Hospital Social Work Self-Efficacy Scale (HSWSE) and the social work field students' self-efficacy ratings in a public hospital. Holden, Cuzzi, Spitzer et al. (1997) further studied the psychometric properties of the HSWSE in a partial replication study of students and hospital social workers. A self-efficacy scale was then developed for caretakers of asthmatic children (Holden, Wade, Mitchell, Ewart & Islam, 1998) extending this line of inquiry. Holden, Barker, Meenaghan and Rosenberg (1999) subsequently developed a measure of student research self-efficacy in social work education, which did not lend itself to this study.

Olsen, Allen, and Azzi-Lessing (1996) reported on risk assessment of substance abuse families that included a subscale of parental self-efficacy. Pearlmutter (1999) provided a review of self-efficacy in relation to organizational change leadership. The only other study of self-efficacy in social work prior to 2000 confused Rotter's internal locus of control (1966) with self-efficacy and was not considered useful to the present study (Kunz & Kalil, 1999). Because self-efficacy is considered situation and task and/or domain specific, the self-efficacy measures reviewed were not useful for child welfare employees.

The first known study of self-efficacy and employee turnover in social work was completed by Ellett (1995). His study attempted to examine the role of self-efficacy motivation and persistence (a consequence of the strength of self-efficacy beliefs) and their relationships to employee *intents to leave employment in child welfare*, general work morale, and job satisfaction. Respondents with low self-efficacy scores indicated high intentions to leave employment in child welfare. The first study of self-efficacy and *employee retention* in social work was a two-state study by Ellett (2000), which is the focus of this article. More recently, Ellett, Ellett, and Rugutt (2003) completed a large, statewide, mixed methods study of self-efficacy and child welfare employee retention and turnover.

Strengthening personal and organizational factors that contribute to the retention of child welfare staff is an important professional and organizational concern. Self-efficacy theory and research are rich, but relatively untapped resources, for studies of employee retention in child welfare. This study was designed to explore how the self-efficacy beliefs of child welfare staff are related to their intentions to remain employed. Establishing linkages between these variables was considered to have important implications for practice, theory development, and future research.

PURPOSE

This study was designed to examine linkages between a theoretically grounded personal/psychological variable, self-efficacy, and child welfare staffs' expressed intentions to remain employed in public child welfare. The purpose of this study was four-fold to:

1. develop new measures of: (a) employee intent to remain (employed); and (b) self-efficacy beliefs specific to child welfare job tasks and work motivation;
2. examine the initial psychometric qualities (validity and reliability) of these new measures;
3. explore empirical linkages between elements of self-efficacy beliefs and employees' intentions to remain employed in child welfare; and
4. discuss implications of the theoretical base and findings from the study for future practice, theory development, and future research.

Given the deep conceptual and research bases of self-efficacy theory, the core hypothesis framing this study was as follows: *There is a statistically significant, positive relationship between the strength of child welfare staff members' self-reported self-efficacy beliefs and their intentions to remain employed in child welfare.*

METHODOLOGY

Sample

All professional level public child welfare staff in the states of Arkansas and Louisiana were included in the study. The total population for the study from the two participating states was 2,140 professional level child welfare staff (1,359 in Louisiana and 781 in Arkansas).

Measures

Self-Efficacy Assessment–Social Work (SEA-SW). This measure operationalized the theoretical construct of self-efficacy reflected in social cognitive theory as described by Bandura (1997). A pool of self-efficacy work task items was developed giving close consideration to tenants of self-efficacy theory (e.g., generality or specificity of work-related tasks). Seventeen of the 20 items generated for the SEA-SW were child welfare work task statements and three items (#s 2, 5, and 12) were statements of motivation and persistence to accomplish work tasks. The final SEA-SW consisted of 19 items that were responded to using the following stem: *The strength of my personal beliefs in my capability to*: (item statement). The response scale was a four-point, forced-choice Likert scale ranging from: 1 = Weak to 4 = Very Strong. The possible score range for the total SEA-SW was 20 to 80. The SEA-SW items and response format are included in the Appendix.

Intent to Remain Employed–Child Welfare (IRE-CW). The Intent to Remain Employed-Child Welfare (IRE-CW) measure consisted of 6 original items developed for this study and three items from a prior study of intent to leave employment in child welfare (Ellett, 1995). *There was no existing measure to assess child welfare employees' intentions to remain employed in child welfare at the time of this study.* The IRE-CW measure represents an alternative to more traditionally used measures in studies of employee turnover in the helping professions that focus on personal/work environment stress factors that contribute to employee turnover and burnout [e.g., Maslach Burnout Inventory developed by Maslach & Jackson, (1986)].

The IRE-CW measure used a four-point, forced choice Likert response format ranging from 1 = Strongly Disagree to 4 = Strongly Agree resulting in a possible score range of 9 to 36. Items numbers 3, 5 and 7 asked respondents about their intentions to leave child welfare employment and were reverse coded for subsequent data analyses. The nine items developed to operationalize child welfare employees' intentions to remain employed in child welfare (IRE-CW) are included in the Appendix. An expert panel review for face and content validation was completed in January 2000 for both measures used in the study.

Social Desirability Index. Four items selected from the work of Crowne and Marlowe (1964) were included in the study along with the other items. These items were included to check on the possibility of participants' responding to the self report measures in a socially desirable manner. These items were: (a) *At times I have wished that something bad would happen to someone I disliked*; (b) *I have sometimes taken unfair advantage of another person*; (c) *I sometimes feel resentful when I don't get my way*; and (d) *I am sometimes irritated by people who ask favors of me*. The same four-point Likert disagreement/agreement scale was used to respond to these items as to the other items. The total social desirability index score ranged from 4 to 16.

Data Collection Procedures

Data for the study were collected in February 2000 by administering a survey packet to all professional level child welfare staff in Arkansas and Louisiana through their respective state offices. Individual paper and pencil packets with return postage envelopes were prepared, packaged and sent to each parish/county/district office within each of the participating states. Individual survey packets included: (a) a cover letter describing state agency approval of and purpose of the study, request for participation, and instructions, (b) the study measures, reflected on an electronically scannable response form, (c) a demographic information form and (d) a self-addressed return postage envelope. Participants were informed about how/why they were selected for the study and advised that all information would be collected in a manner that would maintain participant anonymity and the confidentiality of responses. Time lines for completing the instrument packet (two weeks) were detailed, and procedures for mailing the completed response forms to the researcher were described. Two follow-up reminders were e-mailed to all professional level child welfare staff granting, two, one-week extensions.

Data Analysis Procedures

A variety of quantitative analyses were completed on the survey data. These included:

1. summaries of descriptive statistics (frequencies and percentages) for characteristics of respondents by each state and for the total sample (demographic items);
2. descriptive statistics (means and standard deviations) for items of each measure by each state;
3. principal components analyses of each measure to empirically identify measurement dimensions;
4. descriptive statistics for each factored measurement variable;
5. reliability analyses of the measures for the two-state sample (Cronbach Alphas);
6. bivariate (Pearson product moment) correlations between the self-efficacy measurement subscales (independent variables) and the dependent variable (IRE-CW) to test the core research hypothesis, and between the self efficacy scales, the IRE-CW and the four-item social desirability index.

Data for each of the measures used in the study were analyzed in a series of principal components analysis (PCA) procedures to identify the nature of latent constructs measured (#3 above). Since each of the measures was originally designed for the study, a series of exploratory analyses was completed for the total sample of respondents (n = 941), using PCA procedures and orthogonal rotation of extracted components. For each measure, unconstrained solutions to extract as many components as possible, using the default option of only retaining components that explained at least 1.00% of the total item variance, were followed by iteratively extracting and rotating from one to multiple components. Item/component loadings, scree plots, and variance accounted for by components identified in the various solutions were used to arrive at a final dimensional structure for each measure. The goal in each analysis was to arrive at solutions containing the fewest meaningful components relative to the total variance explained by the particular solution. Negatively worded items were re-coded before these analyses to ease interpretation of item/component/loadings and the interpretation of measurement dimensions. The minimum item/component loading for retaining an item was set at .33. If an item loaded on more than one component, the item was retained on a component only if the difference between the two highest item communalities (squared loadings) exceeded .20.

RESULTS

Descriptive Statistics for Demographics

The complete survey packet described in the methodology section was administered to 2,140 child welfare staff in Louisiana and Arkansas. Only five surveys were considered unusable and were deleted due to excessive missing data. Completed surveys were received from 946 participants (44.2%) representing child welfare staff at all levels within their agencies. The percentage return rates were 41.36% for Louisiana to 45.7% for Arkansas. The final data file with useable responses available for analysis was 941 cases. Descriptive statistics (sample sizes, frequencies, means and standard deviations) were computed on all demographic variables and for each survey measure item. It is beyond the scope of this article to describe all of these results in detail. However those considered of particular interest are noted here.

For the total sample of respondents, 83% were female and 16.7% male with 58.2% of all participants over age 40. By ethnicity, percentages of responses were as follows: 65.3% white, 31.9% African American, and 2.8% other. Percentages of responses by age were 16.7% 30 years or younger, 25.0% between 31 and 40, and 58.2% older than 40 years of age. The major difference between states in the age category, was that 42.6% of Arkansas respondents were 35 years of age and younger, while 44.2% of those responding in Louisiana were between the ages of 46 and 56. Respondents' educational levels included 3% with less than a college Degree. The vast majority of respondents (68.8%) held a baccalaureate degree, and 27.7% with a master's degree. Interestingly, when comparing results for the two states, a considerably larger percentage of staff had master's degrees in Louisiana (40.0%) than in Arkansas (8.7%). Also of note, 8.1% of respondents in Arkansas reported less than a bachelor degree compared to 0.4% in Louisiana. The Bachelor of Social Work represented the most often reported undergraduate degree type (29.8%), with sociology second (15.4%), then psychology

(13.5%). The remaining 41.3% had other undergraduate degrees, and 67.9% of those who reported a master's degree held MSWs.

Length of employment for the total sample was as follows: 1-3 years = 27.0%, 4-9 years = 24.6%, 10-19 years = 22.6 and 20 + years = 22.3%. Perhaps the most noticeable difference when comparing findings for the two states was that 45.8% of Arkansas respondents had 3 years or less child welfare experience compared to 18.9% of Louisiana respondents. Conversely, 34% of Louisiana respondents had 20 or more years experience in child welfare contrasted to 6.6% of those in Arkansas. A detailed summary of descriptive statistics for the sample can be found in Ellett (2000).

Descriptive Statistics for Measures

For the total sample, and the Intent to Remain Employed (IRE) measure, the highest item mean was 3.10 for item # 5 (not actively seeking other employment), and the lowest mean was 2.30 for item # 2 (remain even if offered position outside child welfare with higher salary). Four of the nine IRE item means were lower than the scale mid point. For the total sample on the Self-Efficacy measure, the highest mean was 3.31 for item # 2 (expend energy and effort to accomplish task) and the lowest mean was 2.65 for item # 16 (influence own career opportunities). Twelve of the 20 item means exceeded 3.00, indicating relatively strong self-efficacy beliefs about work tasks. A detailed summary of descriptive statistics for the study measures can be found in Ellett (2000).

Principal Components Analyses (PCA) of the Study Measures

Intent to Remain Employed-Child Welfare (IRE-CW) Measure. Table 1 presents a summary of item communalities and item/component loadings for the PCA analysis of the Intent to Remain Employed (IRE) in child welfare measure. The communalities shown are sums of the squared item/component loadings for each item. The eigen value shown is the sum of all item communalities for an extracted component. The total variance explained is the eigen value divided by the total number of items comprising the measure. All nine of the measurement items were retained in this one-component solution. The item/component loadings ranged from .54 (Item #9) to .76 (item #s 1 and 5). Loadings for six of the nine items approached or exceeded .70. This one-dimensional

TABLE 1. Summary of Item Communalities and Component Loadings for a Uni-Dimensional Solution for the Intent to Remain Employed Measure (n = 941)

Item Number[a]	Communality	Item/Component Loading[b]
1.	.58	**.76**
2.	.50	**.71**
3.	.48	**.69**
4.	.44	**.66**
5.	.58	**.76**
6.	.37	**.61**
7.	.55	**.74**
8.	.56	**.75**
9.	.29	**.54**
Eigen Value	4.36	
% of Variance	48.46	

Note. [a] Item Numbers can be cross-referenced with item statements included in Appendix B.
[b] Item/Component loadings are correlations.

solution accounted for 48.46% of the total item variance. No other dimension was identified in a subsequent multiple component solution. Thus, the Intent to Remain measure was used in subsequent correlation analyses as a one-dimensional measure of employee's intentions to remain employed in CW. The acronym developed for this variable was IRE (Intent to Remain Employed).

Self-Efficacy Assessment-Social Work (SEA-SW) Measure. Data for the self-efficacy measure for the total sample were also analyzed using unconstrained and multiple component PCA solutions with orthogonal rotations. Table 2 summarizes item/component loadings (correlations) for the two-component solution of the self-efficacy measure. The first component was defined by 11 items and accounted for 24.24% of the variance in the solution. Item/component loadings for items retained on this dimension varied from .50 (item # 7) to .70 (item # 9). This dimension was termed Efficacy for Work Tasks (ETSK). Eight items with loadings ranging from .48 (item # 15) to .69 (item # 19) were retained on the second component. This dimension accounted for 18.83% of the total item variance and was termed Efficacy Motivation (EMOT). Collectively

TABLE 2. Summary of Item Communalities and Factor Loadings for a Two-Factor Solution for the Self-Efficacy Beliefs Measure (n = 941)

		Item/Factor Loadings[b]	
Item #[a]	Communalities	Factor I	Factor II
1.	.46	**.65**[c]	.19
2.	.32	.24	**.51**
3.	.47	**.67**	.15
4.	.41	**.55**	.33
5.	.38	.31	**.53**
6.	.41	**.57**	.30
7.	.37	**.50**	.35
8.	.44	**.64**	.18
9.	.51	**.70**	.14
10.	.29	.41	.35
11.	.48	**.64**	.27
12.	.45	.37	**.56**
13.	.37	**.61**	.33
14.	.43	**.59**	.28
15.	.35	.34	**.48**
16.	.35	.19	**.56**
17.	.38	**.57**	.24
18.	.59	.05	**.77**
19.	.44	.21	**.69**
20.	.52	.32	**.65**
Eigen Values	8.61	4.85	3.77
% Variance Explained	43.07	24.24	18.83

Notes. [a] Item Numbers can be cross-referenced with item statements included in Appendix A. [b] Item/Factor loadings are correlations. [c] Bolded numbers indicate final item/factor locations

in this analysis, 19 of 20 efficacy items were retained and the two-component solution accounted for a total of 43.07% of the variance in the data. The correlation between the two self-efficacy components was .69 ($p < .001$).

Reliability Analyses

Data for each of the empirically derived dimensions of the study measures were examined for internal consistency reliability. Cronbach

Alpha reliability procedures were used for each measurement dimension with the entire sample of respondents (n = 941). For the total sample, these reliability coefficients were: IRE = .86; ETSK = .87; EMOT = .81.

Bivariate Correlations Among Factored Dimensions of the Study Measures

Pearson product moment correlation coefficients were computed among all subscales of the study measures to examine interrelationships among the subscales, and to test the core research hypothesis framing the study. The bivariate correlations between the dependent variable, Intent to Remain Employed (IRE) and the independent variables (subscales of the self-efficacy measure) for the entire sample (n = 941) were: IRE with ETSK, r = .17; IRE with EMOT, r = .32. These correlations were positive, in the predicted direction, somewhat moderate in magnitude, and statistically significant ($p < .0001$).

Correlations between the IRE measure and the two self-efficacy dimensions were also computed separately for the total samples of child welfare staff in each state. For the Louisiana sample these correlations were: IRE with ETSK, r = .17; IRE with EMOT, r = .32. For the Arkansas sample these correlations were: IRE with ETSK, r = .20; IRE with EMOT, r = .35. All of these correlations were statistically significant ($p < .001$). These results show a replication of the general relationship between employees' intentions to remain employed in child welfare and dimensions of self-efficacy across the two states. When similar correlations were computed for a sub sample of only caseworker respondents with less than three years of employment in child welfare, these correlations slightly increased in magnitude. These findings provide support for the major hypothesis of the study that predicted statistically significant and positive relationships between child welfare employee's intentions to remain employed in child welfare and the strength of their self-efficacy beliefs related to professional, job-related tasks.

Responses to the study variables showed little influence of social desirability on participants' responses. The correlations between social desirability and the self-efficacy dimensions were ETSK with social desirability (r = .21) and EMOT with social desirability (r = .20). The correlation between this index and the IRE was .03. These results show only 4% common variance between the two dimensions of self-efficacy measured and the index of social desirability of responses and less than 1% shared variance between the social desirability index and the IRE measure.

DISCUSSION AND IMPLICATIONS OF THE FINDINGS

At the time it was completed in spring of 2000, this study was the largest known study of employee retention in child welfare. The findings of the study have implications for understanding the self-efficacy construct within social-cognitive theory and for social work practice in child welfare. The study emanated from the research literature and professional concerns in child welfare pertaining to the important need to study professional child welfare staff to explore factors influencing those who choose to remain in this complex and challenging work environment. Much of the extant literature has focused on trying to understand child welfare employee turnover from a job stress and psychological burnout perspective. This study was framed from an alternative perspective and a research design was developed to better understand personal factors, specifically self-efficacy, predictive of child welfare employees' intentions to remain employed in child welfare. Self-efficacy was derived from the prior conceptual and empirical work of Bandura (1977, 1978, 1986, 1997). The working hypothesis for the study was that *there is a statistically significant, positive relationship between the strength of child welfare staff members' self-reported self-efficacy beliefs and their intentions to remain employed in child welfare*. The results of the study confirmed this hypothesis and replicated this general relationship across two states.

Two new measures were developed for use in the study: one, an index of child welfare employees' intentions to remain employed; and two, a measure of self-efficacy beliefs about core child welfare work tasks. Both of these new measures yielded empirically defined and reliable measurement dimensions for the samples studied. The self-efficacy measure that evolved from the analyses reflected two dimensions of self-efficacy in child welfare settings: (a) Efficacy Work Tasks, and (b) Efficacy Motivation. The Intent to Remain Employed measure demonstrated a one-dimensional structure. As originally hypothesized, employees' perceptions of both dimensions of self-efficacy were positively related to their expressed intentions to remain employed in child welfare. These relationships, while statistically significant, were somewhat moderate in magnitude. The core findings of the study have a variety of implications for practice, theory development, and future research in child welfare. These are addressed in the sections that follow.

Implications for Social Work Practice

The utility of self-efficacy theory and research in understanding child welfare practice, work environments, and retention seems obvious. Development of self-efficacy is critical to child welfare employees' motivation and persistence to develop requisite child welfare knowledge, skills and abilities (KSAs) within this challenging and complex work environment. Workers that develop competence and confidence, will be more likely to experience success with clients and satisfaction with their work (Bandura, 1997), and two recent statewide studies of child welfare workers in California (McElroy, 2002) and Georgia (Ellett et al., 2003) also found this to be the case.

Schools of social work have an important role in developing social work KSAs in their graduates that are needed for effective child welfare practice. The combination of social work courses and field education provides educators opportunities to strengthen self-efficacy beliefs of students by modeling successful practices, making class/field assignments that expand student knowledge and skills through enactive mastery experiences (success), and providing verbal persuasion and emotional supports through a variety of means such as internships, role playing, videotaped observations and analyses, attending to experienced guest speakers, completing case assessments and analyses, structured feedback, actual court observations and/or demonstrations, and so on.

According to Bandura (1997), outcome expectancy is the individual's belief that particular thoughts and actions will lead to expected results. Efficacy expectation is the belief that one has the capability to accomplish a particular task. Both efficacy expectations and efficacy outcome expectancies contribute to personal motivation and persistence to accomplish tasks. A large meta-analysis of 114 studies by Stajkovic and Luthan, (1998) found that self-efficacy was an important predictor of work-related performance. Thus, within the complex and challenging child welfare environment, strengthening self-efficacy beliefs of child welfare staff becomes an important practice concern. Consistent with core tenants of self-efficacy theory, organizations that reward valued accomplishments strengthen employees' self-efficacy beliefs about their capabilities to accomplish assigned tasks and their actions to achieve organizational goals, particularly if employees view their efforts and outcomes as worthwhile.

Translating self-efficacy theory into practice also has important implications for supervision in child welfare. Perhaps the most time consuming and important responsibility child welfare supervisors have is enhancing the development of the core knowledge, skills and abilities (KSAs) that caseworkers need for competent and effective child welfare practice. It takes approximately two years for new caseworkers with no child welfare experience to acquire the KSAs to be able to work independently (Louisiana Work Group, 2000). Close task and quality clinical supervision is especially important to clients assigned to new caseworkers who are learning on the job about the life altering decisions that are made in their cases. In offices with high employee turnover, it is likely that one or more employees in a supervisor's unit are new employees, which creates many stresses and demands on the supervisor for close case consultation. The findings of this study suggest that supervisors who take the time to develop and strengthen caseworkers' self-efficacy beliefs are likely to strengthen employee retention, and thus the quality of services provided to clients that caseworkers serve.

Self-efficacy theory can provide the basis for quality supervision in child welfare. Bandura (1997) identifies four sources of developing and strengthening self-efficacy beliefs. Each of these sources has implications for the various, important roles that supervisors can play in developing employees' belief systems, strengthening their motivation, persistence, and job competence. One source of self-efficacy beliefs is learning through *vicarious experiences*. Thus, the role model that supervisors represent as they work with children and families is a rich observational learning resource for caseworkers they supervise. For example, supervisors can provide vicarious learning opportunities by making home visits with a new worker and demonstrating effective client engagement and interviewing skills. Another source of developing and strengthening self-efficacy beliefs is *verbal persuasion*. Thus, supporting and encouraging workers that they can be successful in performing difficult child welfare tasks, such as preparing a case for court, or testifying in court, are important means of strengthening self-efficacy beliefs.

A third source of self-efficacy is learning through *enactive mastery experience* (actual task success). Bandura describes this source as having the strongest effects on strengthening self-efficacy beliefs. Thus, supervisors who assign tasks to caseworkers commensurate with their capabilities, can enable enactive mastery experiences by helping caseworkers be successful in their work. This is an especially important resource for supervisors in their supervision and mentoring of workers because when workers have successful experiences with clients, they are likely to also experience positive *physiological and affective states*, (e.g., sense of accomplishment, pride in one's work, pleased that they made a difference), a fourth, important source of strengthening self-efficacy beliefs. In addition, developing self-efficacy is a generative process that moves from simple to more complex tasks as these are mastered over time (Maddux, 1999). Thus, supervisors would be well advised to not overload new staff with a large number of complex cases and to work closely with new staff one step at a time.

The four sources of self-efficacy beliefs can singularly, or in combination have either positive or negative effects on individuals. If, for example, a new worker is assigned tasks that are far too difficult (enactive mastery experiences), has few opportunities to observe successful practices by colleagues and supervisors (vicarious experiences), receives little feedback, praise and encouragement (verbal persuasion), the affective components of self-efficacy beliefs will be predictably weak (physiological/affective states), and the employee may then leave employment in child welfare. When these elements all work positively in concert, an employee's self-efficacy beliefs are strengthened and the employee's intentions to remain employed are strengthened as well. This scenario, that integrates self-efficacy beliefs with child welfare practice and employee retention, is supported by the empirical findings in this study and subsequent studies (Ellett et al., 2003; McElroy, 2002).

Implications for Theory and Future Research

The results of this study also have implications for theory development on several levels, and for future research as well. The findings clearly show empirical linkages between child welfare employees' self-efficacy beliefs and their intentions to remain employed in child welfare. Although self-efficacy has been studied extensively in education and psychology, studies of self-efficacy in social work are relatively new, and few have been completed that have attempted to understand self-efficacy within the organizational context (Pearlmutter, 1998). Self-efficacy has been used in research and evaluation studies in social work education programs (Cuzzi et al., 1997; Holden, Anastas, & Meenaghan, 2003; Holden, Barker et al., 1999; Holden, Meenaghan, Anastas, & Mettrey, 2002; Pertrovich, 2004) and in studies of parenting (Coleman, 2000), domestic violence (Danis, 2002); and substance abuse (Kranz, 2003; Olsen, Allen, & Azzi-Lessing, 1996).

The social-cognitive conception of self-efficacy beliefs reflected in the work of Bandura (1978, 1986, 1997) and others has been extended to the child welfare context in this study. According to Bandura, individuals with strong self-efficacy beliefs are highly motivated and persistent in the pursuit of attainment of goals, particularly when they encounter barriers and obstacles to goal attainment. In addition, those with strong efficacy beliefs persist in the face of failure to accomplish goals. Given the difficult and often stressful work environment in which child welfare staff function, the results reported here that positively link the strength of self-efficacy to employees' intentions to remain in child welfare, extend social-cognitive theory into the actual practice setting. The findings also extend the nomological network (Cronbach & Meehl, 1955) and explanatory power of self-efficacy theory to yet another applied setting.

The principal components analysis of the self-efficacy measure clearly identified two statistically independent measurement dimensions (orthogonal rotation of components). The first dimension reflected self-efficacy beliefs about specific work tasks, and the second dimension reflected self-efficacy beliefs pertaining to motivation and persistence to accomplish selected job-related outcomes. The identification of these two measurement dimensions is conceptually and operationally consistent with Bandura's (1997) discussion of self-efficacy beliefs, associated behavioral outcomes, and theory of triadic, reciprocal causation. Consistent with current self-efficacy theoretical conceptions, the two self-efficacy measurement dimensions (tasks and motivation/persistence) were rather strongly and positively related ($r = .69$, $p < .001$). Thus, the findings of this study continue to document the utility of the self-efficacy construct in explaining a wide variety of human behaviors in professional contexts (Bandura, 1978; Holden, 1991; Pajares, 1996; Tschannen-Moran, Hoy, & Hoy, 1998). The correlations between the self-efficacy measure and the intent to remain employed measure provide criterion-related validity evidence for these efficacy measures specifically designed for use in child welfare contexts. They are a starting point for the development of a larger nomological net (Cronbach & Meehl, 1955) from which a more general theory of employee intentions to remain employed (or self-efficacy theory) might emerge.

The measures developed for this study demonstrated reasonable reliability for this particular sample of respondents. While providing some support for construct validity, the findings from the various principal components analyses completed suggest that these measures could be somewhat improved by additional item development and refining the content of the items so the dimensions would account for increasing amounts of variance in the data. As they currently exist, the self-efficacy and intent to remain employed measures continuous can be recommended for use in future research. But as with all measures, improvement in both validity and reliability is an ongoing research concern.

There is an ongoing concern in social-cognitive theory and research about the importance of clearly developing conceptual and operational definitions of the constructs measured. Maddux (1999) has made the argument that key constructs addressed by social-cognitive theory, such as self-efficacy, self-regulation, locus of control, reasoned action and others, share many similarities that are at times confused by language. According to Maddux, "a major source of confusion is that the social-cognitive perspective has a large number of different words but a relatively small number of different ideas. Theorists and researchers need to resist the urge to add words that do not add ideas because doing so will probably add confusion" (p. 34).

At the same time, many different measures of social-cognitive constructs such as self-efficacy exist, which makes research on social-cognitive theory variables challenging and at times confusing. For example, various instruments to measure self-efficacy beliefs have used a variety of response formats such as: "How much confidence do you have that you can . . . ?" "How strongly do you believe you can?" "How strong is your belief that you can?" "The strength of my personal beliefs in my capability to . . . is . . . ," "I feel competent that I can . . . ," and so on. Bandura (1997) has made recommendations about preferred response scales to measure self-efficacy beliefs. However, many different response formats have appeared in the self-efficacy research literature. Thus, there is a continuing need in self-efficacy research in child welfare, and in other contexts as well, to take great care in aligning conceptual and operational definitions of self-efficacy within various contexts. Future theory development in self-efficacy is inextricably interrelated to the logic and quality of operational measures.

In this study, as much as 13% of the variance in child welfare employees' intentions to remain employed was accounted for by elements of self-efficacy beliefs. While this may not appear to be a large percentage of variance accounted for by the combination of these factors, it is considered important when considering the many other factors that contribute to employees' intentions to remain employed in child welfare. For example, financial, personal/social and professional incentives, geographic location, proximity to nearby relatives/family, general levels of satisfaction and dissatisfaction with the community in which one lives, and a host of other factors also undoubtedly contribute to child welfare employee's intentions to remain employed. Thus, accounting for 9% of the variation in intentions to remain employed in child welfare, as was done in this two-state, large sample study, is considered an important, as well as a rather robust statistical finding.

This study was part of the first known study of employee's *intentions to remain employed* in Child Welfare settings using quantitative methods (Ellett, 2000). Consistent with calls for the use of mixed methodologies (quantitative and qualitative), future research in this general line of inquiry might well profit from the use of mixed methods. The quantitative findings, while supporting the research hypothesis, leave some gaps in knowledge that may well be important to fill to further our understanding of personal and organizational factors contributing to persistence in employment in child welfare settings.

One strategy that might be pursued in future research, is to identify statistical outliers in the quantitative data and/or comparison groups of employees with the largest contrasting differences using the variables explored. For example, using the survey data to contrast groups with the highest and lowest reported self-efficacy scores, and cross-tabbing these groups with the strongest and weakest reported intentions to remain employed might be one strategy to identify unique groups for follow-up qualitative research (e.g., individual and focus group interviews, direct observation, participant observation). This mixed methods approach could go a long way in adding explanatory power to the quantitative findings in studies like this and in other studies as well. Knowing that groups *statistically differ* is an important research concern (quantitative findings). But understanding at a more personal level *why* groups differ using qualitative methods extends group differences to a deeper level of understanding. This strategy has been previously used with considerable success in prior statewide studies of personnel needs in child welfare (Ellett, 1995).

The findings also provide conceptual and empirical linkages that can be used to better understand what *intentions to remain employed* really means, and what might influence such intentions. Future studies might, for example, explore linkages of this intention variable to a host of other personal and organizational factors (e.g., personality factors, stress tolerance, general work knowledge, administrative leadership styles, political context factors, organizational culture, human caring, quality of supervision, and so on). As each of these is identified as making a contribution to employee's intentions to persist and remain employed in child welfare, a more general theory of intention, and perhaps holding power of the child welfare organization might emerge. The study reported here represents one step to move in this direction. Future studies, using multiple measures of some of these additional variables, might well lead to a broader understanding of the meaning and complexities of professionals who persist in child welfare, and the organizational characteristics that enhance employee's efforts and persistence, and subsequently that reduce turnover. Ultimately, future research of self-efficacy, employee retention and other personal and organizational variables would focus on how these variables interact to influence client outcomes in child welfare. This study is one step in this direction.

REFERENCES

Aber, J.L. (1983). Social policy issues in the prevention of burnout: a case study. In Faber, B. (Eds.), *Stress and burnout in the human service professions* (pp. 213-226). New York, NY: Pergamon Press.

American Public Human Services Association, (2001). *Report from the child welfare workforce survey: State and county data and findings.* Washington, DC: Author.

American Public Human Services Association. (2005). *Report from the 2004 child welfare workforce survey: State agency findings.* Washington, DC: Author.

Anderson, D.G. (2000). Coping strategies and burnout among veteran child protection workers. *Child Abuse & Neglect, 24*(6), 839-848.

Bandura, A. (1977). *Social learning theory.* Englewood Cliffs, NJ: Prentice Hall.

Bandura, A. (1978). Reflections on self-efficacy. In S. Rachman (Ed.), *Advances in behavior research and therapy, 1,* (pp. 237-269). Oxford: Pergamon.

Bandura, A. (1986). *Social foundations of thought and action: A social cognitive theory.* Englewood Cliffs, NJ: Prentice Hall.

Bandura, A. (1997). *Self-efficacy: The exercise of control.* New York: W.H. Freeman & CO.

Bandura, A., Adams, N.E., & Beyer, J. (1977). Cognitive processes mediating behavioral change. *Journal of Personality and Social Psychology, 35,* 125-130.

Brown, J.K., Chavkin, N.F. & Peterson, V. (2002). Tracking process and outcome results of BSW students' preparing for public child welfare practice: Lessons learned. *Journal of Health and Social Policy, 15*(3/5), 105-116.

Cicero-Reese, B., & Black, P.N. (1997). *Child welfare workers who remain on the job: Why they don't quit.* Paper Present at the Annual Program Meeting of the National Association of Social Workers, Baltimore, MD.

Coleman, P.K. (2000). Parenting self-efficacy among mothers of school-age children: Conceptualization, measurement and correlates. *Family Relations, 49,* 13-24.

Collins, P. (1994). Does mentorship among social workers make a difference? An empirical investigation of career outcomes. *Social Work, 39*(4), (pp. 413-419).

Cronbach, L.J., & Meehl (1955). Construct validity in psychological tests. *Psychological Bulletin, 53,* 281-302.

Crowne, D.P., & Marlowe, D. (1964). *The approval motive.* New York, NY: Wiley.

Cuzzi, L., Holden, G., Rosenberg, G., & Chernack, P. (1996). A pilot study of field work rotations vs. Year long placements for social work students in a public hospital. *Professional Social Work Education and Health Care, 24*(1/2), 73-91.

Danis, F. (2002). Factors that influence domestic violence practice self-efficacy: Implications for social work education. Paper presented at the Annual Program Meeting of the Council of Social Work Education. Nashville, TN.

Dickinson, N.S., & Perry, R.E. (2002). Factors influencing the retention of specially educated public child welfare workers . *Journal of Health & Social Policy, 15*(3/4), 89-103.

Drake, B., & Yadama, G. (1996). A structural equation model of burnout and job exit among child protective services workers. *Social Work Research, 20*(3), 179-187.

Ellett, A.J. (2000). *Human Caring, Self-efficacy Beliefs, and Professional Organizational Culture Correlates of Employee Retention in Child Welfare.* Unpublished doctoral dissertation, Louisiana State University, Baton Rouge.

Ellett, A.J., Ellett, C.D., & Rugutt, J.K. (2003). *A study of personal and organizational factors contributing to employee retention and turnover in child welfare in Georgia: Final project report.* Athens, GA: University of Georgia School of Social Work.

Ellett, A.J., & Leighninger, L. (in press). What happened? An historical analysis of de-professionalization of child welfare.

Ellett, C.D. (1995). *A study of professional personnel needs: Vol. 1.* Baton Rouge, LA: Office of Research and Economic Development, Louisiana State University.

Ellett, C.D., & Ellett, A.J., (1997). Statewide study of child welfare personnel factors: Who stays, who leaves, who cares?. In Martin, T., & Miah, M. (Eds.) A national child welfare challenge: Creating partnerships to strengthen families and children. *Proceedings of the National Conference on Child Welfare.* Carbondale, IL: Southern Illinois University.

Fryer, G.E., Miyoshi, T.J., & Thomas, P.J. (1989). The relationship of child protection worker attitudes to attrition from the field. *Child Abuse and Neglect, 13*(3), 345-350.

Gansle, K.A., & Ellett, A.J. (2002). Collaboration in child welfare preparation: Evaluating a higher education/state agency model. *Journal of Health & Social Policy, 15*(3/4), 69-88.

Harrison, S.G. (1995). Exploration of factors related to intent to leave among child welfare caseworkers. Doctoral dissertation, Ohio State University. *Dissertation Abstracts International, The Humanities and Social Sciences, 56*, 9, (1996) 3744-A.

Helfgott, K. (1991). *Staffing the child welfare agency: Recruitment and retention.* Washington, D.C.: Child Welfare League of America, Inc.

Holden, G. (1991). The relationship of the self-efficacy appraisals to subsequent health related outcomes: A meta-analysis. *Social Work in Health Care, 16*(1), 53-93.

Holden, G., Anastas, J. & Meenaghan, T. (2003). Determining attainment of the EPAS foundation program objectives: Evidence for the use of self-efficacy as an outcome. *Journal of Social Work Education, 39*, 4250440.

Holden, G., Barker, K., Meenaghan, T., & Rosenberg, G. (1999). Research on self-efficacy: A new possibility for educational outcomes assessment. *Journal of Social Work Education, 35*(3), 463-476.

Holden, G., Cuzzi, L., Rutter, S., Rosenberg, G. & Chernack, P. (1996). The hospital social work self-efficacy scale: Initial development. *Research on Social Work Practice, 6*(3), 353-365.

Holden, G., Cuzzi, L., Spitzer, W., Rutter, S., Rosenberg, G., Chernack, P. & Rosenberg, G. (1997). The hospital social work self-efficacy scale: A partial replication and extension. *Health and Social Work 22*(4), 256-263.

Holden, G., Meenaghan, T., Anastas, J. & Mettrey, G. (2002). Outcomes of social work education: The case for social work self-efficacy. *Journal of Social Work Education, 38*(1), 115-133.

Holden, G., Wade, S.L., Mitchell, H., Ewartz, C., & Islarm, S. (1998). Caretaker expectations and the management of pediatric asthma in the inner city: A scale development study. Social Work Research, 22(1), 51-59.

Hopkins, K.M., Mudrick, N.R. & Rudolph, C.S. (1999). Impact of university/agency partnerships in child welfare on organizations, workers and work activities. *Child Welfare,78*(6), 749-773.

Jayaratne, S., & Chess, W. (1984 a). Factors associated with job satisfaction and turnover among child welfare workers. In J. Laird & a. Hartman (Eds.), *A handbook of child welfare: Context, knowledge, and practice* (pp. 760-766). New York, NY: The Free Press.

Jayaratne, S., & Chess, W. (1984 b). Job satisfaction, burnout, and turnover: A national study. *Social Work, 29*(5), 448-453.

Johnson, S. (1999). *College choice: Psychological factors influencing postsecondary aspirations and expectations of ninth-grade students*. Unpublished doctoral dissertation, Louisiana State University, Baton Rouge.

Jones, L. (2002). A follow-up of a Title IV-E program's graduates' retention rates in a public child welfare agency. *Journal of Health & Social Policy, 15*(3-4), 39-51.

Kern, H., McFadden, T., Baumann, D., & Law, J. (1993). *Caseworker study part I: Burnout and turnover*. Austin: TX. Department of Protective and Regularity Services.

Kranz, K.M. (2003). Development of the alcohol and other drug self-efficacy scale. *Research on Social Work Practice, 13*(6), 724-741.

Kunz, J. & Kalil, A. (1999). Self-esteem, self-efficacy and welfare use. *Social Work Research, 23*(2), 119-126.

Lewandowski, C.A. (1998). Retention outcomes of a public child welfare long-term training program. *Professional Development: International Journal of Continuing Social Work Education, 1*, 38-46.

Lewandoski, C.A. (2003). Organizational factors contributing to worker frustration: The precursor to burnout. *Journal of Sociology and Social Welfare, 30*(4), 175-185.

Liederman, D. (1998). *A critical look a the child welfare system caseworker turnover*. Child Welfare League of America. Washington, DC.

Louisiana Work Group, (2000). *Louisiana OCS Job Study*. Document in preparation for presentation to the state Civil Service to upgrade all OCS child welfare professional level positions, Baton Rouge, LA. Author.

Maddux, J.E. (1999). Expectancies and the social-cognitive perspective: Basic principles, processes, and variables. In Kirsch, I. (Ed). *How expectancies shape experience*. Washington, DC: American Psychological Association.

Maslach, C., & Jackson, S.E. (1986). *Maslach Burnout Inventory: Manual*. Palo Alto, CA: Consulting Psychologists Press, Inc.

McElroy, K.L. (2002). *Factors associate with high self-efficacy among California's public child welfare workers*. Unpublished master thesis, California State University, Los Angles.

McMahon, J. (1999). Turnover in child welfare. *Practice Notes for North Carolina Child Welfare Workers, 4*(3), 1-3, 8.

Mor Barak, M.E., Nissly, J.A. & Levin, A. (2001). Antecedents to retention and turnover among child welfare, social work, and other human service employees: What can we learn from past research? A review and metanalysis. *Social Service Review, 75*(4), 625-661.

Olsen, L.J., Allen, D., & Azzi-Lesing, L. (1996). Assessing risk in families affected by substance abuse. *Child abuse and Neglect, 20*(9), 833-842.

Pajares, F. (1996). Self-efficacy beliefs in academic settings. *Review of Educational Research, 66*(4), 543-578.

Pearlmutter, S. (1999). Self-efficacy and organizational change leadership. *Administration in Social Work, 22*(3), 23-38.

Petrovick, A. (2004). Teaching Notes: Using self-efficacy theory in social work teaching. *Journal of Social Work Education, 40*(3), 429-443.

Reagh, R. (1994). Public child welfare professionals: Those who stay. *Journal of Sociology and Social Welfare, 21*(3), 69-78.

Robin, S.C. & Hollister, C.D, (2002). Career paths and contributions of four cohorts of IV-E funded MSW child welfare graduates. *Journal of Health and Social Policy, 15*(3/5), 53-67.

Rycraft, J. (1994). The party isn't over: The agency role in the retention of public child welfare caseworkers. *Social Work, 39*(1), 75-80.

Rycus, J. & Hughes, R. (1994). *Child welfare competencies.* Columbus, OH: Institute for Human Services.

Samantrai, K. (1992). Factors in the decision to leave: Retaining social workers with MSWs in public child welfare. *Social Work, 37*(5), 454-458.

Scully, R. (1983). The work-setting support group: A means of preventing burnout. In B. Farber (Ed.), *Stress and burnout in the human service professions* (pp 188-197). New York, NY: Pergamon Press.

Söderfeldt, M., Söderfeldt, B., & Warg, L.E. (1995). Burnout in social work. *Social Work, 40*(5), 638-46.

Stajkovic, AlD. & Luthans, F. (1998). Self-efficacy and work-related performance: A meta-analysis. *Psychological Bulletin, 124*(2) 240-261.

Tett, R., and Meyer J. (1993). Job satisfaction, organizational commitment, turnover intention, and turnover: Path analysis based on meta-analytic findings. *Personnel Psychology, 46*, 259-293.

Tschannen-Moran, M., Hoy, A.W., & Hoy, W.K. (1998). Teacher efficacy: Its meaning and measure. *Review of Educational Research, 68*(2), 202-248.

United States Government Accounting Office (1995). *Child welfare: Complex needs strain capacity to provide services.* Washington, DC: Author.

U. S. General Accounting Office, (2003). *Child welfare: HHS could play a greater role in helping child welfare agencies recruit and retain staff.* Washington, DC: Author.

Vinokur-Kaplan, D. (1987). Where did they go? A national follow-up of child welfare trainees. *Child Welfare, 67*(5), 411-421.

Vinokur-Kaplan, D. (1991). Job satisfaction among social workers in public and voluntary child welfare agencies. *Child Welfare, 70*(1), 81-91.

Zimmerman, B.J. (1989). A social cognitive view of self-regulated social academic learning. *Journal of Educational Psychology, 81*, 329-339.

doi:10.1300/J394v04n03_04

APPENDIX A

SELF-EFFICACY ASSESSMENT–SOCIAL WORK

Directions

This part of the survey requests that you make judgments about the ***strength of your personal beliefs in your capabilities to organize and carry out tasks to successfully accomplish outcomes in child welfare***. In assessing the strengths of your personal beliefs about each task, consider your abilities in the work context, job roles and responsibilities, available resources, agency support, current policies, help from colleagues, and so on. For each item, fill in the corresponding number.

1 = *Weak* (W) 2 = *Somewhat Strong* (SS) 3 = *Strong* (S) 4 = *Very Strong* (VS)

	The strength of my personal beliefs in my capability to:	**W**	**SS**	**S**	**VS**
1.	use assessment skills in decision making about child safety is...	1	2	3	4
2.	regularly expend the energy and effort to accomplish work tasks is...	1	2	3	4
3.	effectively use interviewing skills is...	1	2	3	4
4.	engage individuals in strengths and problem identification is...	1	2	3	4
5.	remain motivated and persist in overcoming difficult or uncertain obstacles to accomplish outcomes for clients is...	1	2	3	4
6.	provide social work treatment interventions with families whose children are in foster care is...	1	2	3	4
7.	simultaneously implement reunification and adoption permanency goals (concurrent planning) is...	1	2	3	4
8.	analyze and synthesize information required for legal actions in child welfare cases is...	1	2	3	4
9.	be an effective witness in child welfare court hearings is...	1	2	3	4
10.	communicate critical written information in a way that is well organized and clear is...	1	2	3	4
11.	work effectively with family members in child neglect cases is...	1	2	3	4
12.	rebound and persist after failures in my efforts to accomplish work goals is...	1	2	3	4
13.	assist children in working through separation from their family members is...	1	2	3	4
14.	accurately assess parenting capability is...	1	2	3	4
15.	effectively work with clients and co-workers in a culturally sensitive manner is...	1	2	3	4
16.	influence my career opportunities in the child welfare organization in which I work is...	1	2	3	4
17.	work with child sexual abuse victims, non-offending parents and sexual perpetrators is...	1	2	3	4
18.	work effectively within the structure of my state organization is...	1	2	3	4
19.	work collaboratively with staff from other community agencies is...	1	2	3	4
20.	interpret and apply agency policies in my job assignment is...	1	2	3	4

APPENDIX B

INTENT TO REMAIN EMPLOYED–CHILD WELFARE

Directions

This section of the survey asks you to make a series of judgements about your personal attitudes and beliefs. The best answer is the one that most accurately reflects your personal views and opinions. Please respond to each statement using the scale provided below. Fill in one number for each item that best corresponds to the strength of your disagreement or agreement using a **# 2 pencil.**

SCALE: 1 = Strongly Disagree (SD) 2 = Disagree (D) 3 = Agree (A)
4 = Strongly Agree (SA)

		SD	D	A	SA
1.	I intend to remain in child welfare as my long-term professional career.	1	2	3	4
2.	I will remain in child welfare even though I might be offered a position outside of child welfare with a higher salary.	1	2	3	4
3.	I would leave child welfare work tomorrow if I was offered a job for the same salary but with less stress.	1	2	3	4
4.	The personal and professional benefits outweigh the difficulties and frustrations of working in child welfare.	1	2	3	4
5.	I am actively seeking other employment.	1	2	3	4
6.	I feel the personal and professional gratification of working in child welfare to be greater than those in other professions.	1	2	3	4
7.	I frequently think about quitting my job.	1	2	3	4
8.	I am committed to working in child welfare even though it can be quite stressful at times.	1	2	3	4
9.	My intention to remain employed in child welfare is stronger than that of most of my colleagues.	1	2	3	4

Correlates of Secondary Traumatic Stress in Child Protective Services Workers

Brian E. Bride, PhD
Jenny L. Jones, PhD
Samuel A. MacMaster, PhD

SUMMARY. The purpose of this study was to add to the limited research on secondary traumatic stress in child welfare by investigating correlates of secondary traumatic stress (STS) in child protective services workers. Specifically, we examined the relationship between levels of STS in CPS professionals and personal history of trauma, peer and administrative support, intent to remain employed in child welfare, professional experience, and size of caseload. This study documents the existence of secondary traumatic stress in the population and the relationship between levels of secondary traumatic stress in CPS professionals and the group of potential correlates: personal history of trauma in the past year and lifetime, peer support, administrative support, intent to remain employed in child welfare, professional experience, and size of caseload. doi:10.1300/J394v04n03_05 *[Article copies available for a fee from The Haworth Document Delivery Service: 1-800-HAWORTH. E-mail address: <docdelivery@haworthpress.com> Website: <http://www.HaworthPress.com> © 2007 by The Haworth Press, Inc. All rights reserved.]*

Brian E. Bride is affiliated with the University of Georgia.
Jenny L. Jones and Samuel A. MacMaster are affiliated with the University of Tennessee.

[Haworth co-indexing entry note]: "Correlates of Secondary Traumatic Stress in Child Protective Services Workers." Bride, Brian E., Jenny L. Jones, and Samuel A. MacMaster. Co-published simultaneously in the *Journal of Evidence-Based Social Work* (The Haworth Press, Inc.) Vol. 4, No. 3/4, 2007, pp. 69-80; and: *Developing an Empirically Based Practice Inititative: A Case Study in CPS Supervision* (ed: Jenny L. Jones, and Paul Sundet) The Haworth Press, 2007, pp. 69-80. Single or multiple copies of this article are available for a fee from The Haworth Document Delivery Service [1-800-HAWORTH, 9:00 a.m. - 5:00 p.m. (EST). E-mail address: docdelivery@haworthpress.com].

Available online at http://jebsw.haworthpress.com

doi:10.1300/J394v04n03_05

KEYWORDS. Child protective services, secondary traumatic stress, burnout, employee retention

CORRELATES OF SECONDARY TRAUMATIC STRESS IN CHILD WELFARE

The psychological effects of direct exposure to traumatic events such as childhood abuse, criminal victimization, natural disaster, and war and terrorism are well documented. Dozens of books and hundreds of scientific articles have been published documenting the nature and dynamics of traumatic stress (Wilson & Raphael, 1993). The majority of those reports, however, focus solely on those who were directly traumatized (Figley, 1999). It has become increasingly apparent that the effects of traumatic events extend beyond those directly affected. The term secondary traumatic stress has been used to refer to the observation that those who come into continued close contact with trauma survivors, including human service professionals, may experience considerable emotional disruption and may become indirect victims of the trauma themselves (Figley, 1995). Consequently, secondary traumatic stress is becoming viewed as an occupational hazard of providing direct services to traumatized populations (Figley, 1999; Munroe et al., 1995; Pearlman, 1999).

The negative effects of secondary exposure to a traumatic event are nearly identical to those of primary exposure (Figley, 1999). Chrestman (1999) notes that secondary traumatization may include symptoms observed in persons directly exposed to trauma such as: intrusive imagery related to the client's traumatic disclosures, avoidant responses, physiological arousal, distressing emotions, and functional impairment. In addition to these PTSD-like symptoms, the consequences of providing services to traumatized populations may also include "significant disruptions in one's sense of meaning, connection, identity, and world view, as well as in one's affect tolerance, psychological needs, beliefs about self and other, interpersonal relationships, and sensory memory" (Pearlman & Saakvitne, 1995, p. 151). First explicated by McCann and Pearlman (1990), this transformation in cognitive schemas and belief systems resulting from empathic engagement with clients' traumatic experiences has been termed vicarious traumatization. Secondary traumatic stress and vicarious traumatization both refer to the same phenomenon, however, the STS concept focuses primarily on symptomology, while the concept of vicarious traumatization focuses on meaning and adaptation (Pearlman & Saakvitne, 1995b).

Despite a rapidly expanding literature on secondary and vicarious traumatization, there remains a relative dearth of research into this area. Bride (2004) conducted a review of 15 studies of secondary traumatic stress in individuals who provide psychosocial services to traumatized populations, and concluded that the empirical evidence provides support for the notion that individuals who provide psychosocial services are at risk of experiencing symptoms of traumatic stress, disrupted cognitive schema, and general psychological distress as a result of their work with traumatized populations. However, the severity of these experiences varied across studies from mild symptom levels (Brady, Guy, Poelstra, & Brokaw, 1999; Chrestman, 1999; Follette, Polusny, & Milbeck, 1994; Ortlepp & Friedman, 2002; Steed & Bicknell, 2001) to levels similar to those of persons in outpatient treatment for PTSD (Arvay & Uhleman, 1996), and only a subset of study participants reported symptoms. There is some evidence that younger service professionals may be at increased risk (Arvay & Uhleman, 1996; Ghahramanlou & Brodbeck, 2000), however, this may have less to do with age and more to do with the development of coping mechanisms that comes with increased experience. That is, younger professionals are likely to be newer to the field and less like to have had the opportunity to develop protective strategies to deal with the difficulties of working with traumatized populations. In regards to the influence of exposure to traumatized populations on levels of secondary traumatic stress, the length of experience providing general psychosocial services seems to have less influence on symptomatology than the length of experience specifically providing trauma services. In addition, it appears that level of exposure to traumatized clients is more important than length of exposure in that higher proportions of traumatized clients on caseloads (Chrestman, 1999; Kassam-Adams, 1999; Schauben & Frazier, 1995), and higher proportion of time spent in trauma-related clinical activities are more predictive of secondary trauma symptoms (Brady et al., 1999). Although there has been speculation that providing services to traumatized children places providers at higher risk for secondary traumatic stress as compared to work with adults, the empirical evidence does not bear this out (Brady et al., 1999; Meldrum, King, & Spooner, 2002). However, results of several studies indicate that a personal trauma history, particularly in childhood, is a significant risk factor (Ghahramanlou & Brodbeck, 2000; Kassam-Adams, 1999; Nelson-Gardell & Harris, 2003; Pearlman & Mac Ian, 1995). Further, the use of social supports and positive coping strategies appear to be associated with lower levels of symptomatology (Follette et al., 1994; Schauben & Frazier, 1995). It should be noted, however, that the findings summarized above should be viewed with caution, as findings were generally mixed in each of the specific areas reviewed.

Secondary Traumatic Stress and Child Welfare

With two exceptions noted below, the articles included in the review cited above reported primarily on psychotherapists and sexual assault counselors. Several authors have noted that CPS professionals are particularly at risk for the development of STS symptoms given their daily contact with physically, sexually, and emotionally abused children (Bell, Kulkarni, & Dalton, 2003; Horwitz, 1998). Despite the fact that CPS workers are logically at risk for STS, only two studies have been published that examine STS in this population. The first study found that CPS workers experienced greater psychological distress that the general population, and many reported distress levels greater than those reported by typical outpatient mental health clients (Cornille & Myers, 1999; Meyers & Cornille, 2002). In addition, longer tenure in the CPS field was associated with higher levels of STS and working more than 40 hours per week was associated with higher levels of STS. The second study of STS in child welfare was reported by Nelson-Gardell and Harris (2003) who conducted a study of 166 child welfare staff, including child protection workers, supervisors and managers who took part in an evaluation of a STS training program in two states. Participants completed a demographic questionnaire, the Childhood Trauma Questionnaire (Bernstein & Fink, 1998), and the Compassion Fatigue Self Test for Psychotherapists (Figley, 1995). Consistent with several studies in other populations, their findings suggest that a personal history of childhood trauma increases a child welfare worker's risk of STS. More specifically, a combination of more than one type of childhood trauma presents the greatest risk for vulnerability to STS, with emotional abuse and neglect being the strongest predictors of STS.

The purpose of this study is to add to the limited research on STS in child welfare by investigating correlates of secondary traumatic stress in child protective services workers. Specifically, we examined the relationship between levels of secondary traumatic stress in CPS professionals and personal history of trauma in the past year and lifetime, peer support, administrative support, intent to remain employed in child welfare, professional experience, and size of caseload.

METHODOLOGY

Data Collection

Data was collected by means of a web-based survey. The e-mail addresses of all CPS case managers and supervisors in the state of Tennessee were obtained from the Tennessee Department of Children's Services. An e-mail with a brief description of the study, the use of the data, the risks and benefits involved in participating in the study, and the confidentiality of the data was sent to all CPS workers. The e-mail provided participants with a link to the URL containing the survey instruments, as well as login and password information required to access the survey. No identifying information was solicited, although participants were asked to provide a unique identifier consisting of the first two letters of their mother's maiden name, the last two digits of their year of birth, and the last two digits of their social security number. Two additional e-mails were sent at one week intervals requesting participation in the study. The Website containing the survey instruments was shut down three weeks following the initial e-mail.

Instrumentation

Demographic Information Questionnaire (DIQ). The DIQ is a 27-item survey constructed specifically for this study. Items were designed to gather standard demographic information (age, gender, ethnicity, salary, education, etc.) as well as information regarding specifics of their job (i.e., position, length of time in position, size of caseload, etc.) (Table 1).

Intent to Remain Employed–Child Welfare (IRE-CW). The IRE-CW (Ellet & Millar, 2001) contains 9 items and uses a four-point Likert response format ranging from *strongly disagree* to *strongly agree* to assess respondents' intention to leave child welfare employment. The IRE-CW is based on a conceptual definition of employee intent to remain employed that is derived from an understanding of personal, psychological, and work context factors and encompasses cognitive, affective, and behavioral elements. The IRE-CW has been found to have factor validity and internal consistency (coefficient alpha = .86) (Ellett & Millar, 2001).

Secondary Traumatic Stress Scale (STSS). Designed to measure work-related secondary traumatic stress in human service professionals, the STSS (Bride, Robinson, Yegidis, & Figley, 2004) is comprised of three subscales (Intrusion, Avoidance, and Arousal) that are congruent with the PTSD symptom clusters as delineated in the DSM-IV-TR (APA, 2000). Respondents indicate how frequently they experienced each of 17 symptoms during the previous week using a five-choice, Likert-type response format ranging from *never* to *very often.* The STSS has demonstrated evidence of convergent, discriminant, and factor validity, as well as Cronbach alpha levels for each subscale and the entire scale as follows: Total Scale = .93, Intrusion = .80, Avoidance = .87, and Arousal, = .83 (Bride et al., 2004).

Professional Organizational Culture Questionnaire–Social Work (POCQ-SW). The POCQ-SW (Ellett & Millar, 2001) is a 26-item instrument designed to assess three dimensions of organizational culture by means of the following subscales: Administrative Support, Professional Sharing and Support, and Professional Commitment. Investigation of internal consistency resulted in coefficient alphas of .92 for Administrative Support, .83 for Professional Sharing and Support, and .83 for Vision/Professionalism/Commitment. Further, evidence supported the factor validity of the instrument (Ellett & Millar, 2001).

RESULTS

A total of 333 CPS professionals in the state of Tennessee were contacted via E-mail to participate in this study, of which 187 completed surveys were received representing a 56% response rate. Respondents were primarily female (83%) with a mean age of approximately 37. Three-quarters of respondents identified their ethnicity as Caucasian (76.1%), with the remainder identifying as African-American (20.7%) or Other (3.2%). Most (87.2%) indicated their highest educational level was a bachelors degree with only 11.7% reporting having a masters degree and 2 (1.1%) reporting a high school degree as their highest educational level. 81.9% of respondents were in case management positions and 18.1% identified as supervisors.

Respondent's mean scores on the STSS, POC, and IRE-CW are presented in Table 2. Scores on the STSS and its subscales represent moderate levels of secondary trauma in the sample. Of course this represents an aggregate mean. More telling is the fact that 92% of respondents reported experiencing at least one STS symptom at least "occasionally" in

TABLE 1. Demographic and Professional Characteristics of Respondents

	n	X	S.D.	%
Age	187	36.95	11.04	
Experience (yrs)	277	16.15	9.59	
Gender				
Female	156			83.0
Male	32			17.0
Ethnicity				
Caucasian	143			76.1
African American	39			20.7
Other	6			3.2
Highest Educational Level				
High School	2			1.1
Bachelors	164			87.2
Masters	22			11.7
Position				
Case Manager	154			81.9
Supervisor	34			18.1

Note: Percentages may total more than 100% due to rounding error.

TABLE 2. Summary Scores on the STSS, POC, and IRE-CW

	n	$\bar{x}$	SD
Secondary Traumatic Stress Scale			
Intrusion Subscale	187	10.97	4.07
Avoidance Subscale	187	15.64	5.98
Arousal Subscale	187	11.58	4.22
Total Score	187	38.20	13.38
Professional Organizational Culture Questionnaire			
Administrative Support Subscale	179	31.55	6.84
Professional Sharing and Support	186	21.69	4.08
Vision and Professional Commitment	184	24.48	3.67
Intent to Remain Employed–Child Welfare Scale	186	23.30	5.68

the week preceding the survey and 59% reported experiencing one or more STS symptoms "often" during the same period. Further, 34% of respondents met the core criteria for work related PTSD (APA, 2000) as indicated by experiencing at least one intrusion, three avoidance, and two arousal symptoms "often" in the prior week.

Table 3 displays the bivariate correlations (Pearson's *r*) between secondary traumatic stress levels as measured by the total STSS scores and correlates of interest. Of the seven correlations tested, four were found to be statistically significant at an alpha level of less than .05. The magnitudes of two of these correlations were relatively small; STS symptoms were negatively correlated with peer support ($r = -.145$) and positively correlated with caseload size ($r = .171$). That is, higher levels of peer support were associated with lower levels of STS symptoms and higher caseloads were associated with increased STS symptoms. A somewhat stronger correlation was found between STS symptoms and a personal history of trauma ($r = .247$), although no relationship was found with a recent trauma history. The strongest correlation ($r = -.388$) was found between STS symptoms and intent to remain employed, suggesting that higher levels of STS symptoms are associated with a desire to leave the field.

DISCUSSION

This study adds to the limited research on secondary traumatic in child welfare by providing data on the existence, and correlates of, secondary traumatic stress in child protective services workers. Specifically, we were able to begin to document the existence of secondary

Table 3. Bivariate Correlations with the STSS Total Score

	n	*r*
Past year trauma history	174	NS
Lifetime trauma history	177	.247**
Peer support	185	–.145*
Administrative support	178	NS
Intent to remain employed	185	–.388**
Professional experience (yrs)	187	NS
Caseload size	187	.171*

Note: NS = not significant, * = $p < .05$, ** = $p < .01$.

traumatic stress in the population, as moderate levels of secondary trauma were found in the sample as a whole, and more than a third of the sample met the core criteria for work related PTSD. Of course, this data is only suggestive of similarly high prevalence rates, but they are consistent with the notion that child welfare workers are at particularly high risk for developing secondary traumatic stress symptoms given the incidence of the traumatic situations the children that they work with experience coupled with the possibilities of a less than supportive work environment. The present study does not allow formal testing of this notion, though further study is clearly warranted.

Perhaps the most interesting findings presented in this paper are the documentation of the relationship between levels of secondary traumatic stress in CPS professionals and the group of potential correlates: personal history of trauma in the past year and lifetime, peer support, administrative support, intent to remain employed in child welfare, professional experience, and size of caseload. The study was able to find statistically significant correlations between secondary traumatic stress levels as measured by the total STSS scores and four of the correlates of interest: peer support, caseload size, personal history of trauma, and intent to remain employed, and a lack of relationship with a personal history of recent trauma, administrative support, and professional experience.

These results are consistent with the literature, yet are of particular importance within the realm of child welfare as the employer can potentially impact three of the four correlations through interventions. Clearly support for these interventions is outside the scope of the study, however, the results suggest the possibility that by decreasing caseload size and cultivating opportunities for peer support individual workers may experience an amelioration of secondary trauma. Interestingly, peer support rather than administrative support was found to be significant, which is further suggestive of the type of support that needs to be cultivated. While intent to remain employed is as much a possible outcome of STS, it too may be reduced through awareness and interventions directed at decreasing its impact. Given the concerns about worker turnover in child welfare, this appears to be an area that can be directly addressed by child welfare agencies. The fourth correlate is interesting in that a history of personal trauma was significantly correlated with STS rather than recent personal trauma suggesting that there may be a predisposing factor to this phenomenon.

There are some obvious limitations to the data presented here. First, as the data is drawn from convenience sampling procedures, the responses in this study may not be representative of all child welfare workers.

Heightening this concern is that fact that the participation rate for the survey was only 56%. Many CPS workers chose not to be involved in the project. This may have occurred for a variety of reasons: difficulties in maintaining contact with workers, concerns on the part of the worker regarding their confidentiality, and/or lack of investment in the topic due to not having had experienced secondary trauma. Second, the sample size (n = 187), while adequate for the purposes of this study, clearly limits our ability to draw reliable conclusions to the entire population of child welfare workers. However, given the descriptive focus of the analyses presented, the sample size is appropriate to the study purpose. Actual prevalence rates and relationships to other variables are outside of the scope of this study. Future research efforts may want to test such questions in a more scientific manner.

REFERENCES

American Psychiatric Association (2000). *The diagnostic and statistical manual of mental disorders (4th ed., text revision).* Washington, DC: Author.

Arvay, M.J. & Uhlemann, M.R. (1996). Counsellor stress in the field of trauma: A preliminary study. *Canadian Journal of Counselling, 30*(3), 193-210.

Bell, H., Kulkarni, S., & Dalton, L. (2003). Organizational prevention of vicarious trauma.*Families in Society, 84*, 463-470.

Bernstein, D. & Fink, L. (1998). *Childhood Trauma Questionnaire: A retrospective self-report manual.* San Antonio, TX: The Psychological Corporation

Birck, A. (2001). Secondary traumatization and burnout in professionals working with torture survivors. *Traumatology, 7*(2), Article 2. Retrieved on September 9, 2003, from http://www.fsu.edu/~trauma/art2v7i2.htm

Brady, J.L., Guy, J.D., Poelstra, P.L., & Brokaw, B.F. (1999). Vicarious traumatization, spirituality, and the treatment of sexual abuse survivors: A national survey of women psychotherapists. *Professional Psychology: Research and Practice, 30*, 386-393.

Bride, B.E. (2004). The impact of providing psychosocial services to traumatized populations. *Stress, Trauma, and Crisis: An International Journal, 7*, 29-46.

Bride, B.E., Robinson, M.M., Yegidis, B., & Figley, C.R. (2004). Development and validation of the Secondary Traumatic Stress Scale. *Research on Social Work Practice, 14*, 27-35

Chrestman, K.R. (1999). Secondary exposure to trauma and self reported distress among therapists. In B.H. Stamm (Ed.), *Secondary traumatic stress: Self-care issues for clinicians, researchers, & educators* (2nd ed., pp. 29-36). Lutherville, MD: Sidran Press.

Cornille, T.A. & Myers, T.W. (1999). Secondary traumatic stress among child protective service workers: Prevalence, severity, and predictive factors. *Traumatology, 5*, 1-14.

Ellett, A.J. & Millar, K.I. (2001). *A multi-state study of professional organizational culture: Implications for employee retention and child welfare practice*. Paper presented at the Society for Social Work and Research 5th Annual Conference, Atlanta, Georgia.

Figley, C.R. (Ed.) (1995). *Compassion fatigue: Coping with secondary traumatic stress disorder in those who treat the traumatized.* New York: Brunner/Mazel.

Figley, C.R. (1999). Compassion fatigue: Toward a new understanding of the costs of caring. In B.H. Stamm (Ed.), *Secondary traumatic stress: Self-care issues for clinicians, researchers, & educators* (2nd ed., pp. 3-28). Lutherville, MD: Sidran Press.

Follette, V.M., Polusny, M.M, & Milbeck, K. (1994). Mental health and law enforcement professionals: Trauma history, psychological symptoms, and impact of providing services to child sexual abuse survivors. *Professional Psychology: Research and Practice, 25*, 75-282.

Ghahramanlou, M. & Brodbeck, C. (2000). Predictors of secondary trauma in sexual assault trauma counselors. *International Journal of Emergency Mental Health, 2*, 229-240.

Horwitz, M. (1998). Social worker trauma: Building resilience in child protection social workers. *Smith College Studies in Social Work, 68*, 363-377.

Kassam-Adams, N. (1999). The risks of treating sexual trauma: Stress and secondary trauma in psychotherapists. In B.H. Stamm (Ed.), *Secondary traumatic stress: Self-care issues for clinicians, researchers, & educators* (2nd ed.). Lutherville, MD: Sidran Press.

McCann, I.L. & Pearlmann, L.A. (1990). Vicarious traumatization: A framework for understanding the psychological effects of working with victims. *Journal of Traumatic Stress, 3*, 131-149.

Meldrum, L., King, R., & Spooner, D. (2002). Secondary traumatic stress in case managers working in community mental health services. In C.R. Figley (Ed.), *Treating compassion fatigue* (pp. 85-106). New York: Brunner-Routledge.

Munroe, J.F., Shay, J., Fisher, L., Makary, C., Rapperport, K., & Zimering, R. (1995). Preventing compassion fatigue: A treatment team model. In C.R. Figley (Ed.), *Compassion fatigue: Coping with secondary traumatic stress disorder in those who treat the traumatized.* New York: Brunner/Mazel.

Myers, T.W. & Cornille, T.A. (2002). The trauma of working with traumatized children. In C.R. Figley (Ed.), *Treating compassion fatigue* (pp. 39-55). New York: Brunner-Routledge.

Nelson-Gardell, D. & Harris, D. (2003). Childhood abuse history, secondary traumatic stress, and child welfare workers. *Child Welfare, 82*, 5-26.

Pearlman, L.A. (1999). Self-care for trauma therapists: Ameliorating vicarious traumatization. In B.H. Stamm (Ed.), *Secondary traumatic stress: Self-care issues for clinicians, researchers, & educators* (2nd ed.) (pp. 51-64). Lutherville, MD: Sidran Press.

Pearlman, L.A. & Mac Ian, P.S. (1995). Vicarious traumatization: An empirical study of the effects of trauma work on trauma therapists. *Professional Psychology: Research and Practice, 26*, 558-565.

Pearlmann, L.A. & Saakvitne, K.W. (1995). *Trauma and the therapist: Countertransference and vicarious traumatization in psychotherapy with incest survivors.* New York: W.W. Norton & Company.

Schauben, L.J. & Frazier, P.A. (1995). Vicarious trauma: The effects on female counselors of working with sexual violence survivors. *Psychology of Women Quarterly, 19*, 49-64.

Wilson, J.P. & Raphael, B. (Eds.) (1993). *International handbook of traumatic stress syndromes*. New York: Plenum.

doi:10.1300/J394v04n03_05

Numbers Alone Do Not Tell the Whole Story: A Program Evaluation Designed to Generate Evidence-Based Knowledge and Practice in Child Welfare Supervision

S. Yvette Murphy, PhD, MSW
Judy Goodson, LMSW

SUMMARY. This article presents an overview of a mentoring effort focused on child welfare supervisors. The longitudinal, mixed-methods program evaluation applied to the effort is presented and discussed. Employing a control group and a comparison group of child welfare supervisors across the state of Arkansas, the program evaluation was designed to generate knowledge to support evidence-based practice within the field of child welfare supervision. Although the mentoring effort and program evaluation are still underway, an exploration of the preliminary

---

S. Yvette Murphy is Assistant Professor and Judy Goodson is Title IVE Project Director, University of Arkansas School of Social Work.

Address correspondence to S. Yvette Murphy, PhD, 106 ASUP, Fayetteville, AR 72701 (E-mail: ymurphy@uark.edu).

The authors are grateful for the assistance of Arkansas DCFS staff, Mentoring of Supervisors Project staff, University of Arkansas School of Social Work, and Hornsby Zeller Associates. The Mentoring of Supervisors Project was funded through The Children's Bureau via a grant to the Southern Regional Quality Improvement Center.

[Haworth co-indexing entry note]: "Numbers Alone Do Not Tell the Whole Story: A Program Evaluation Designed to Generate Evidence-Based Knowledge and Practice in Child Welfare Supervision." Murphy, S. Yvette, and Judy Goodson. Co-published simultaneously in the *Journal of Evidence-Based Social Work* (The Haworth Press, Inc.) Vol. 4, No. 3/4, 2007, pp. 81-101; and: *Developing an Empirically Based Practice Inititative: A Case Study in CPS Supervision* (ed: Jenny L. Jones, and Paul Sundet) The Haworth Press, 2007, pp. 81-101. Single or multiple copies of this article are available for a fee from The Haworth Document Delivery Service [1-800-HAWORTH, 9:00 a.m. - 5:00 p.m. (EST). E-mail address: docdelivery@haworthpress.com].

Available online at http://jebsw.haworthpress.com

doi:10.1300/J394v04n03_06

findings reveal valuable lessons with the primary lessons being the need to consider both the process and the outcomes when evaluating program efforts within complex organizational settings such as child welfare.
doi:10.1300/J394v04n03_06 *[Article copies available for a fee from The Haworth Document Delivery Service: 1-800-HAWORTH. E-mail address: <docdelivery@haworthpress.com> Website: <http://www.HaworthPress.com>*

KEYWORDS. Evidence-based practice, program evaluation, child-welfare supervision, process and outcomes, mentoring

INTRODUCTION

In response to criticism of the performance of child welfare agencies, mandates to demonstrate accountability, and sincere desires to promote effective practice, the child welfare system is interested in determining if the interventions and efforts proclaimed as best-practices are indeed achieving specified outcomes. This interest has sparked a need for the type of knowledge that is necessary to inform evidence-based practice (EBP). Evidence-based practice is that which uses scientifically sound knowledge as the basis for making decisions about what one does in day-to-day practice that will be effective within a given context (Roberts & Yeager, 2004). Program evaluations of efforts believed to promote best-practice and to achieve specified outcomes are helpful in generating knowledge to support EBP (McNeece, 2004). To offer assistance in generating such knowledge, the Administration of Children and Families (ACF) Children's Bureau funded five Regional Quality Improvement Centers (QICs) for child protection and adoption services in 2001 and charged the centers with championing efforts to assess the needs, identify knowledge gaps, and improve the quality of child welfare practice. One of the awardees under this effort was the University of Kentucky's College of Social Work, which established the Southern Regional Quality Improvement Center (SR QIC) for Child Protection.

Although the factors that impact the effectiveness of child welfare efforts are multiple and confluent in nature (Pecora, Whittaker, Maluccio, Barth & with Plotnick, 1992), findings from the Southern Regional Quality Improvement Center needs assessment (SR QIC, 2001) reveal that the best-practice efforts relative to child welfare supervision is one area in need of exploration. With a belief in the critical nature of the supervisory relationship on the attainment of numerous outcomes such as job satisfaction, turnover rates of child welfare practitioners and the attainment of positive outcomes on behalf of the children and families the child welfare system serves, and aiming to develop and implement efforts to strengthen the capacity of child welfare programs to achieve specified outcomes, the Arkansas Division of Children and Family Services (DCFS) accepted the challenge to explore best-practice efforts relative to child welfare supervision. DCFS proposed to develop, systematically implement, and evaluate an effort to generate evidence-based knowledge relative to the best-practice claims of child welfare supervision. With mentoring being selected as the primary modality for intervention, the focus of the Arkansas project was "structured casework supervision," and the project effort was titled, Arkansas Mentoring Supervisors Project (AMSP).

Hayward (2004) suggests that sensitivity to context is important when making informed or evidenced-based decisions, and Rosenthal (2004) suggests that the intended purpose of EBP is to improve the process *and* outcome of service efforts and interventions. However, child welfare supervisors often encounter several barriers with respect to implementing such practices. First, although the availability of scientifically generated literature is a prerequisite to a child welfare supervisor's ability to engage in EBP, and, although child welfare supervisors who turn to the literature in such an attempt will find a wealth of suggestions that are based on practice wisdom and experience, Usher (2004) suggests, that child welfare practitioners are not likely to find scientifically generated evidence from which to make decisions about best and effective practice. Second, the new focus within the child welfare arena on outcomes has resulted in diminished attention to the concepts of process and context. Addressing these gaps in literature is crucial because without comprehensive, scientific evidence to assist supervisors from multiple perspectives, that is; in knowing the *outcomes* of a specified effort as well as the *processes* that lead to certain outcomes within a specified context, supervisors are "solely relying on practice wisdom, tradition, or 'common sense'" (McNeece & Thyer, 2004, p. 8). While social work judgment and practice wisdom are not invalid resources, relying solely on such conventions in directing efforts and decisions that have the potential to determine the difference between life and death outcomes for children is unacceptable. Thus, a primary goal of the Arkansas effort is to address this gap in the literature. Although this study has yet to be completed and the findings are preliminary, this article aims to contribute to the literature by presenting potential challenges of generating evidence-based knowledge within the context of the child welfare system, providing an overview of the AMSP effort along with implementation challenges and systemic barriers specific to the effort, sharing preliminary findings of the AMSP effort and discussing lessons learned that hold implications for child welfare practice and research.

Potential Challenges of Generating Scientific Evidence to Support the Practice Efforts of Child Welfare Supervisors

Roberts and Yeager (2004) indicate that, "[s]ocial work has a history related to evidence-based practice dating back to the 1970s and the work of Mullen and Dumpson (1972), Fischer (1973) and Jayaratne and Levy (1979)" (p. 9). Although the contributions of EBP to the field of social work are clearly documented (McNeece & Thyer, 2004; Roberts & Yeager, 2004; Usher, 2004), McNeece and Thyer (2004) suggest that, "adoption of EBP within the profession seems to continue at a slow pace, slower in some areas of practice than others." (p. 8). While not acceptable as an excuse, there are several challenges that may provide insight into why evidence-based literature to support child welfare supervisory practice is limited and not emerging as quickly.

First, for studies to be both helpful and effective in directing practice within the complex culture of the child welfare system, the study design requires the use of complex, often non-traditional, multi-system designs that include mechanisms for ongoing feedback and employ opportunities for both quantitative and qualitative methods (Gleeson, 1992). In spite of the potential benefits, employing complex research designs to support evidence-based practice is often complicated by numerous variables (Rosen, 2003). Other potential challenges relate to what appears at times to be conflicting goals between child welfare administrators, practitioners and researchers, and the ever changing, unstable, nature of the child welfare context. Researchers concerned with systematically implementing efforts and protecting the integrity of the research design often have little tolerance for changes in a design. Although divergent perspectives have historically led to tension among researchers and practitioners, Usher (2004) suggests that attention to the differing perspectives that researchers and human service practitioners have relative to their roles in developing and testing intervention efforts is leading to an emergence of collaborative efforts that are more helpful and responsive to the needs of families.

A second challenge is the cost in both tangible dollars and human resources of creating complex, multi-systems, creative, multi-method designs. Although cost is a factor for most of the concerns within the child welfare system, the exclusion of research- related activities as an allowable expense for one of the largest child welfare funding sources, Title IV-E; makes the challenge to produce scientifically sound research to support EBP more difficult than many other challenges.

Limited access to research data is another limitation. The involuntary nature of the child welfare system coupled with the necessary confidentiality requirements and Internal Review Board protections may present challenges to obtaining data needed for multi-level, non-traditional, multi-method research designs that may favor direct observation of interactions between supervisors, caseworkers, and clients.

Links exist between research, policy and practice with practitioners and policy makers often looking to the literature for answers and ideas. When efforts to sustain feedback loops between research, policy and practice are not systematically supported and maintained, the generation of evidence-based knowledge is often limited or fails to become incorporated into policy and practice (Rosen, 2003). Taking on these challenges, Arkansas' MFSS effort offers a model for (1) strengthening the capacity of supervisors and (2) assessing the best practice efforts of child welfare supervisors for evidence of effectiveness.

PROJECT OVERVIEW

In 1999, Arkansas' Division of Children and Family Services (DCFS) engaged in a federal Child and Family Services Review (CFSR) conducted by the Administration of Children and Families (ACF) Children's Bureau. The review focused primarily on DCFS' performance relative to the outcomes of (1) safety, (2) permanency, and (3) well-being for the children and families in the state. As in the case of every other state, the review resulted in a need for a Program Improvement Plan (PIP). In reviewing the overall findings of the CFSR and aiming to incorporate the findings into the PIP, Arkansas' DCFS observed that the CFSR focused primarily on outcomes with less attention to process. Arkansas believed this to be a major limitation of the review, as without consideration or analysis of the processes that led to such outcomes or the context in which the outcomes were assessed, little help was available in identifying the various factors such as staffing levels, caseload sizes, retention or support needs of field staff that were influencing the outcomes. This limitation prohibited insight or direction about specific processes, or contextual influences that needed attention in order for the outcomes to be achieved. Further observing the absence of evidence-based knowledge to support EBP among child welfare supervisors, Arkansas DCFS conceptualized and proposed the AMSP to SR QIC and established the goals of having a positive impact on child welfare practice, client outcomes, worker commitment and generating evidence relative to the best-practice claims of child welfare supervisory practices.

The Arkansas Mentoring Supervisors Project is a joint project between DCFS, University of Arkansas, Fayetteville and University of Arkansas, Little Rock and the Arkansas Commission on Child Abuse, Rape and Domestic Violence. By developing, systematically implementing, and evaluating a supervisory mentoring effort based upon the best practice suggestions within the literature, the specific aims of the project are to develop a plan to improve the process and outcomes related to child welfare supervision, to track and assess the relationship between specific processes and outcomes; and to support EBP by measuring the intervention and its impact on practice. To achieve these aims, structured and systematically implemented research methods were used. The selected methods hold the capacity to determine whether or not the employed best-practice efforts would produce certain outcomes and, if so, what are the specific processes that led to, hindered, or had no affect on such outcomes.

Overview of Conceptualization

Administration, support and education are the three primary functions of supervision (Kadushin, 1976). A study on the self-perceptions of supervisors found that child welfare supervisors perceive the skill of mentoring to be most valued (Zunz, 1995). However, due to a variety of factors, the past efforts of Arkansas' child welfare supervisors traditionally focused primarily on the administration function with much of the supervisory training and competencies emphasizing administrative duties and tasks and giving minimal attention to the support and education functions essential to mentoring and developing Family Service Workers (FSW). When asked to identify their training and education needs relative to supervisory practice, Arkansas supervisors overwhelmingly reported a need for mentoring with a focus on policy clarification and on-the-job training (SR QIC, 2001).

DCFS based their approach on Social Learning Theory (Bandura, 1977) which suggests social interaction is the vehicle through which learning occurs and the model of parallel process (Williams, 1997) which suggests that patterns tend to repeat themselves across systems and thus emphasizes a dynamic interchange between the supervisor and supervisee along with a structured support element provided via a mentor (Kane, 1991). DCFS conceptualized a learning laboratory approach to executing a mentoring effort that builds upon the instructional, interactional and educational components of the supervisor/supervisee relationship (Munson, 1995; Shulman, 1993). The effort incorporates mechanisms such as structured and regular case reviews, facilitation of self-awareness (Bernatovicz & Barkley, 1995) and training on theories of supervision (Gleeson & Philbin, 1996) to support the systematic implementation of five key concepts of supervision (i.e., structure, regularity, consistency, case orientation, and evaluation) identified by Munson (1995) as supervisory best-practices. Focusing not only on outcomes, but also on the processes that lead to certain outcomes, the conceptual framework for the study suggests that based upon the assumptions of social learning theory (Bandura, 1977), the principles of parallel process (Williams, 1997) and the use of interactional, instructional and educational components, participation in the study will result in a supervisor-mentor relationship that would lead to engagement in certain processes and learning which are in turn passed on to the supervisor-FSW relationship that leads to the FSW employing such learning in their work with client families thereby achieving positive outcomes.

Description of Project

The central focus of the project was the mentoring of child welfare supervisors to improve their supervisory skills. Of particular importance was the shifting of supervisor's primary focus, time and attention from the "non-administrative" functions of supervision to the supervision functions related to support and education (see Kadushin, 1992).

The mentoring of child welfare supervisors in the intervention group consisted of a number of different modalities including regularly scheduled meetings with an experienced mentor, formal classroom training, structured on-the-job training activities (including on-line tutorials), and ongoing field education and mentoring for a two-year period. The supervisors, in turn, were supposed to apply the lessons learned in their mentoring interactions to their interactions with their caseworkers by means of: regularly scheduled face-to-face meetings with their workers, and a comprehensive review of **all** cases on the worker's caseload as opposed to just problematic cases.

Description of the Mentoring Process

The Arkansas Mentoring Supervisors project was developed with intentions of departing from business as usual. To begin this departure, activities such as weekly individual sessions between the mentors and supervisors focused on: implementing weekly individual sessions between the supervisors and FSWs, the implementation of structured case reviews, teaching team building skills, marketing these new roles to others. Other steps included an orientation to the grant proposal and objectives, and provision of support and materials to assist the supervisors in self-evaluation As a part of the process, mentors meet weekly on an individual bases with each supervisor for no less than an hour, facilitated project-wide team meetings and retreats that incorporated educational, supportive and technical assistance components. Although the mentors prepared agendas for individual meetings, space was allowed for supervisors to engage in brainstorming or venting session, with the focus on adaptive coping or solutions. In addition to promoting and supporting the use of the structured case reviews, the mentors facilitated the supervisors' engagement in assessing and addressing the professional needs of their staff and themselves, with a focus on self-care.

The project mentors both had Master of Social Work Degrees and were Licensed Certified Social Workers with numerous years of social work practice and supervisory experience.

Process Challenges

In spite of good intentions and structured efforts to depart from business as usual, the AMSP encountered several challenges and barriers. One barrier was the hesitancy to become engaged among a few supervisors who perceived their selection for mentoring as punishment or as a suggestion that they were poor supervisors.

Time was another challenge. Some supervisors stated time limitations and staffing ratios as the biggest barriers to structured case reviews. For most supervisors, developing mechanisms to enhance the structured case review process, such as utilizing the structured case review form, was the primary expressed interest, and the major focus of the early effort of the educational component.

Distance was a barrier to participation in team meetings for the northern part of the state. The grant proposed monthly team meetings to be done either face-to-face or via compressed video. Technological limitations in some of the more remote areas resulted in poor reception of the compressed video signal, thus the compressed video meetings were discontinued. With distance and technology challenges, the supervisors in the northern part of the state decided to meet every other month, while supervisors in the southern part of the state continued to meet every month.

Although participant supervisors' acceptance of the project varied, most voiced support of the concept behind the effort. However, because of other demands, mainly related to the agency's focus on obtaining accreditation from the Council on Accreditation of Services to Children and Families (COA), supervisors often felt burdened with program expectations. Consequently, for a period of time, many of the supervisor-mentor sessions focused on providing outlets for frustration.

Systemic barriers that lead to low morale, such as a hiring freeze to replace vacant positions, were also encountered. However, regular and ongoing dialogue about the needs among the supervisors, mentors and the state office staff resulted in mechanisms and processes to address some of the systemic barriers.

METHOD

Research Questions and Hypotheses

The primary research question supporting this study is whether participation in the supervisory mentoring effort, which incorporates key processes, accepted as best-practice lead to improvement of key outcomes relative to child welfare practice. The specific hypotheses along with the identified processes and outcomes are as follows:

1. As a result of systematic and structured case consultation, leading to mentoring and improved support, the practice of child welfare workers under the supervision of study participants will show improvement relative to the areas of assessment and intervention as determined by improved worker responses on the Caseworker Survey.
2. As a result of structured casework supervision, leading to enhanced learning, skill development and systematic and structured support, the FSWs of supervisors in the study effort will show improvement in the three specified outcomes for the families they serve as determined by quarterly reports on client outcomes.

3. As a result of structured case supervision leading to an increased sense of supervisory support, increased regularity, standardized content and promotion of clearer understanding of core practice expectations, preventable worker turner among FSW supervised by study participants will improve as determined by the Caseworker Survey and exit interviews.

Participants

The effort began with selecting the intervention group that included child welfare supervisors who had a minimum of one year of child welfare supervisory experience at the beginning of the project and whose primary job was supervising family services workers (FSW) or family service worker trainees (FSWT) who delivered ongoing child protective services. Those who supervised family service workers that carry caseloads consisting only of foster care or investigations were not included in the study group. The comparison group consisted of other supervisors in the state who were identified as having somewhat similar experience as those of the intervention group. As a whole, 40 of the state's 75 counties, representing both rural and metropolitan areas were selected for participation in the project, either as treatment or control counties.

Demographic and Background Characteristics of Participants

Table 1 presents some basic data on the demographic and background characteristics of project participants who completed the first administration of the survey, conducted in August, 2003 at the beginning of the mentoring intervention and analyzed by Hornby Zeller and Associates (Hornby & Zellar, 2005). The table presents information on six characteristics. The first three characteristics (sex, race, and highest level of education completed) are categorical variables for which results are presented in terms of percentage distributions, while the second three (age, number of years in the field of social services, and number of years working for DCFS) are quantitative variables for which results are presented in terms of median years. Data are broken out by type of worker (supervisor vs. caseworker) and treatment status (intervention vs. control).

The data in the table show that gender composition of the samples varies by type of worker and treatment status. Supervisors have higher percentages of females than do caseworkers, and within each class of worker, the intervention group has higher percentages of females than

TABLE 1. Mentoring Supervisors: Participant Demographics

Demographic and Background Characteristics of Intervention and Control Groups, by Type of Worker

	Supervisors		Caseworkers	
Percentages	Intervention	Control	Intervention	Control
Gender				
Male	6.7	11.1	12.1	15.6
Female	93.3	88.9	87.9	84.4
Race				
White	66.7	66.7	51.5	71.1
Black	33.3	33.3	45.5	28.9
Am. Indian	0.0	0.0	3.0	0.0
Highest Educational Level Completed				
HS/GED	0.0	0.0	3.0	6.7
Some College	6.7	0.0	3.0	0.0
Assoc. Degree	0.0	0.0	0.0	0.0
Bach. Degree	66.7	94.4	84.8	88.9
Master's Deg.	26.7	5.6	9.1	4.4
Doctoral Deg.	0.0	0.0	0.0	0.0

	Supervisors		Caseworkers	
Median Years	Intervention	Control	Intervention	Control
Age	46.0	48.5	30.0	36.0
Years in soc. SVCS.	11.9	13.2	4.2	4.3
Years with DCFS	10.4	12.4	2.2	4.3
Sample Sizes	15	18	33	45

does the control group. In terms of racial composition, two-thirds of the supervisors participating in the study were white. Among caseworkers, racial composition varied by group assignment; around 52 percent of the caseworkers in the intervention group were white, compared to 71 percent of the control group. With only a few exceptions, the overwhelming majority of participants in the study have at least a bachelor's degree. Supervisors in the intervention group, however, have the highest percentage of participants with master's degrees (26.7 percent). On average, supervisors were somewhat older than caseworkers, although participants in control counties (regardless of worker type) were somewhat older than their counterparts in intervention counties. In terms of number of years working in the field of social services, supervisors had significantly more experience than did caseworkers, and supervisors in control counties had slightly more experience than their counterparts in intervention counties. As far as specific work experience with DCFS is concerned, supervisors (in general) had more years of experience than did caseworkers, and within each class of worker, participants from control counties had slightly more experience than did their counterparts in intervention counties.

Overall, supervisors in general and supervisors in control counties in particular were the oldest and most experienced participants in the study, although supervisors in intervention counties had the highest levels of formal education. The various groups also differed in terms of their gender and racial composition; although it is by no means clear just how these differences might affect project outcomes.

Research Design

The study evaluation was based upon a quasi-experimental, comparison group, longitudinal design and used both qualitative and quantitative methods. Such a design is viewed as favorable for generating evidence-based knowledge (National Science Foundation, 1997). Since evaluations are most effective to practitioners when they are systematic and ongoing (National Science Foundation, 1997) the evaluation process was structured in three main phases (1) the establishment of baseline data (2) ongoing or formative assessment and (3) an annual/final or summative assessment were structured into the evaluative process. Each one of the phases involved analysis at multiple levels; the supervisory level, the FSW and FSWT level, the client level (client outcomes and satisfaction) and the organizational level (organizational culture and process).

Quantitative Measures: Focus on Outcomes

The quantitative measure focused on outcomes in three main areas. The areas included: (1) FSW practice as measured by self-efficacy, favorable case review, and client satisfaction (2) FSW turn over as defined by preventable turnover rates, and positive assessment of the quality of the office work environment as determined by a measure of professional organizational culture and (3) client outcomes as defined by three specific service outcomes: (1) the percent of initial contact with families within 24 hours in the project counties, (2) the percent of cases with subsequent substantiated maltreatment reports within 6 months of first substantiated report, and (3) the percent of intact families with cases open for ongoing child protection services over 12 months. Data was also collected to compare the characteristics and demographics for the intervention and control groups of the supervisors and the FSW's under their supervision. Data for comparison of the outcomes and group comparisons was obtained through quarterly statistical reports generated by DCFS and the use of a 62-item survey instrument that was developed locally with guidance and assistance from SRQIC research staff. Most of the survey items were taken from the Survey of Professional Child Welfare Staff developed for the Georgia Division of Family and Children Services (Ellett & Ellett, 2002). Other items were tailored specifically to the unique characteristics of the Arkansas project. Separate surveys were developed for the supervisors and caseworkers.

Supervisor Survey

The supervisor survey included five dimensions. The first dimension focused on the various practices that might be used in the supervision of child welfare caseworkers. Responses were measured by means of a Likert-type scale of agreement/disagreement, with the responses aggregated and averaged to produce scores on a "supervision scale." Scale scores could range from zero through five, with higher scores indicating "better supervisory practice."

Second dimension questions were taken from the previously cited Survey of Professional Child Welfare Staff (Ellett & Ellett, 2002) and were intended to measure respondents' intent to remain employed in the field of child welfare. Responses to these items were aggregated to produce a "commitment scale," with higher scores indicating higher levels of commitment to remaining in the field.

Questions from the third dimension were also taken from the Survey of Professional Child Welfare Staff and constitute what Ellett et al. (2002) refers to as a measure of "professional organizational culture." Higher scores on the organizational culture scale indicate more positive assessment of the quality of the office work environment.

The fourth dimension included questions related to a subset of items that constitute what Ellet et al., (2002) refer to as the scale of "efficiency expectations." This scale is designed to assess the respondents' assessments of how effective they can be in producing positive client outcomes. Higher score on this scale indicate a higher level of expectations. Questions on the fifth dimension captured demographic data.

The Caseworker Survey included six dimensions with the items and scales comparable to the Supervisor Survey. The additional dimension included a "self-efficacy scale" (Ellett & Ellett, 2002) designed to assess caseworkers' beliefs about their own abilities to achieve successful outcomes in child welfare.

Qualitative Measures: Focus on Process

Preliminary qualitative data was obtained primarily through reports completed by project mentors and minutes of project meetings and retreats. Final analyses will include information from exit interviews, focus groups and client surveys. The qualitative measures focused on the various processes related to the effort and included a measure of (1) treatment fidelity; that is, the extent to which the actual program components or supervisor behaviors are taking place, (2) Worker Satisfaction, (3) Supervisory Practice; that is achievement of project-specific, individualized, learning objectives, and (4) External Factors that may influence project implementation or research findings such as hiring freezes or legislative changes). The purpose of the qualitative process was to supplement the quantitative aspects of the evaluation and assist in contextualizing and interpreting the quantitative findings by capturing both the numbers (quantitative data) and the stories (qualitative data), to present a fuller, more comprehensive picture of the impact and value of the intervention.

ANALYSIS

The findings reported in this article are preliminary as the study is still in process and all data collected thus far has not been analyzed. For purposes of this article, the preliminary findings that are reported include qualitative data drawn from minutes of project meetings and consistent themes identified from the monthly reports of the mentors. In terms of quantitative data the preliminary findings reported include demographic and benchmark data. Final analysis will pertain to four administrations of quantitative data collected and qualitative material from project meetings and mentor reports over a two and one-half year period. The first two administrations of quantitative data were collected in August, 2003 and March, 2004 with the final two administrations being collected in 2005. The first administration of the focus group data was collected between July, 2003 and December, 2004 with the remaining administrations being collected throughout the project.

RESULTS

Quantitative: Survey Response Rates and Initial Observations

It should be noted that only two administrations of surveys have been administered at this time; consequently, insufficient data is available to report detailed findings. Some descriptive findings were available for the two matched groups to be included in this article.

Fifteen of the 20 intervention supervisors (75%) and 18 of the 30 supervisors (60%) from the control group, completed surveys during the first administration. Of those who responded in the first administration, 10 of 15 intervention supervisors (66.7%) and 17 of the 18 supervisors (94.4%) in the control group completed surveys again in the second administration.

For caseworkers, 36.3 percent of sampled intervention caseworkers and 42.9 percent of sampled control caseworkers completed surveys during the first administration, with follow up survey rates of 36.4 percent and 66.7 percent, respectively. These response rates are of the same order of magnitude as those reported in an analysis of comparable data from the Mississippi project site (Sullivan et al., 2004)

Benchmark scores were high. Responding workers showed a high regard for supervision, a satisfaction with a supportive culture, and, a strong sense of self-efficacy. It is possible for the mentoring intervention to make a difference in these venues, but the already high scores make the task of finding statistically significant differences even more exacting.

Qualitative: Feedback from Project Supervisors and Mentors

Although the qualitative data also have yet to be fully collected and analyzed, common themes in support of the intervention have begun to surface. Statements gleaned from reports done by the mentors indicated DCFS Supervisors saw the increased use of the structured case review as a tool to increase the critical thinking skills of caseworkers. One Supervisor reported, "The structured case review is helpful even on cases I routinely discuss with my staff. In routine discussions, they sometimes forget to tell me details that are important to the overall case." Another Supervisor noted that she "liked the structured case review because it offered a more detailed, written review of the case progress and who is to take what action next." A third Supervisor reported using the structured case review as an opportunity to focus on success, and to plan for quality court presentations. Triaging crisis situations was a productive use of the structured case review noted by yet another Supervisor.

Project Supervisors also reported that caseworkers were seeing the supervisory sessions as growth experiences rather than critical, punitive interactions. Routinely having the workers in closed door sessions in the Supervisor's office allowed the Supervisor to privately discuss issues with workers without raising suspicions and fears of disciplinary action, and allowed corrections to be made without having to progress to documented corrective action.

One Supervisor said she was, "consciously using techniques from the list of supervisory techniques with a trainee." She said focusing on the parallel process was helping with development of this trainee's skills.

Although the Supervisors in this study have faced many systemic challenges, they have acknowledged their leadership roles via parallel process by modeling strengths-based responses. One Supervisor noted that "not focusing on the negative with both her workers and her bosses is helping her be productive. She went on to say, "I get tired of hearing the bad stuff and I know that my supervisors get tired too. Not being negative helps us focus on the current problem."

Observation by mentors reflected increased self-esteem of the Supervisors as evidenced by their heightened verbalizations at quarterly meetings reflecting a mutual sense of respect and trust. A sense of camaraderie was evidenced when the Supervisors said they liked sharing common issues with other Supervisors and enjoyed hearing the thoughts of other Supervisors. The opportunity to share their thoughts and concerns with DCFS executive staff was reported as an added bonus.

A project Supervisor summed her thoughts on the project meetings and retreats when she stated, "The quarterly mentoring meetings and summer retreats have demonstrated knowledge can be free, questions are acceptable, motivation is contagious, and thus the Mentoring Project is an employee friendly, knowledge based environment."

DISCUSSION

Lessons Learned: Implications for Child Welfare Practice and Research

McNeece (2004) indicates that program evaluations are helpful in generating evidence to support "whether or not a program works, under certain conditions" (p. 592). McClintock (2004) goes further to suggest the importance of considering and assessing issues of organizational development when doing program evaluations. Although the study effort is not at the final stage and the results are preliminary, the suggestions of McNeece and McClintock are similar to the valuable lessons learned from the AMSP effort.

Attention to Setting the Stage

Organizational literature talks much about the challenges related to organizational change (McClintock, 2004). Policy changes relative to the Adoption and Safe Families Act (ASFA) passed and revised by Congress in the 1990's along with feedback from Federal Reviews have resulted in the child welfare system experiencing more changes in the last decade or so than it has its entire history. While most agree that such changes are positive, in that the changes were needed, the magnitude of change and the negative experience with change made it difficult for some supervisors to embrace the AMSP effort. For example, it took six months to develop rapport and trust among the stakeholders. Thus, an important lesson learned relative to implementing change efforts within the context of child welfare is to take the time to set the stage and acknowledge the natural feelings and anxieties that those undergoing the change may have. While this lesson sounds simplistic, it is one that is rarely considered when implementing efforts or interventions within the child welfare system. It is important that this process be systematically and purposefully incorporated into intervention efforts and that efforts towards change are directed at all levels of the system and not just the supervision or direct-service level.

The Numbers Do Not Tell the Entire Story

The purpose of evidence-based knowledge is to guide the best practice efforts of practitioners. It is widely accepted that knowledge to support EBP needs to be of use to the practitioner, accessible and scientifically generated. Yet, many efforts to generate such knowledge culminate in traditional, quantitative designs that focus solely on outcomes, are absent of detail relative to process, and do not consider the organizational context. Experience with this project has already revealed that finding a statistically significant difference as a result of the mentoring intervention could be a challenge. Baseline scores of respondent workers were high, and in many cases systemic challenges such as staff turnover, a hiring freeze, and Project Supervisors assuming caseloads have altered the amount of time supervisors could devote to meeting with Mentors and learning new skills. While the quantitative findings are too preliminary to draw specific conclusions, the preliminary qualitative findings suggest the process has proven valuable to Project Supervisors in ways that were not measured on the survey. Thus, perhaps the most significant preliminary lesson learned from the AMSP effort is that numbers alone do not tell the entire story. When clear relationships between outcomes and intervention efforts are not determined, are practitioners then to discard the intervention? Or, should practitioners and researchers be encouraged to explore and consider other intervening variables related to the process and to the context in which the intervention occurred? Social work practice is grounded in an ecological perspective and has historically been concerned with the concepts of process and context. Yet, efforts to generate evidence, based solely upon outcomes, has the propensity for excluding or not giving full consideration to contextual and process factors such as high caseloads, vacant positions and hiring freezes that carry a significant influence on outcomes.

Evidence-based practice is essential and needed and as Yeager (2004) suggests, given the value of human life, "[c]learly a link exists between program evaluation [and] health and human services" (p. 652). However, we must be cautious of making decisions *only* in terms of outcomes. This lesson holds implications for efforts to generate evidence-based knowledge as well as efforts to evaluate and use such knowledge.

To be most helpful to practitioners, scientifically generated knowledge needs to offer more than the "what," that is whether an effort or intervention produced a certain outcome. Process related information; that is, information that speaks to the "how" along with consideration of the contextual interactions that occur within and between multiple levels of the system is needed. For example, the CFSR is thorough in its efforts to examine the outcomes of whether or not a worker-supervisor staffing occurred. However, the lack of attention to context and process limits the instrument's ability to offer guidance to supervisors and practitioners about how; that is, what processes result in the effectiveness of the achieved outcome. In addition, the absence of analysis of process and contextual factors limits the ability of the knowledge to be fully replicated and fully assessed.

The reality is, outcome measurement is appropriately a sound and preferable foundation for making practice decisions, but it is not the only factor that needs to be considered. To fully embrace the definition of EBP, that is practice which is based upon the most effective and comprehensive, scientifically-generated means, it is important that researchers and practitioners work together to generate knowledge from a "both/and" perspective to research, that is, a perspective that equally considers the numbers and the stories, that is both outcomes and process when aiming to generate knowledge that will guide EBP. In addition, the success of a mentoring, or any other intervention effort, is closely tied to the context or environment in which the effort is implemented and assessed. Thus it is also important to consider context. This is especially important within child welfare as its context embodies characteristics such as: complexity, constant change, complex policies, involuntary client base, a crisis oriented nature, and over-burdened staff who are charged with carrying the enormous responsibility of protecting the lives of children. While the field of health and practice among the medical profession and others that are leaders in EBP may carry many similar challenges, the fact that the context of child welfare offers additional, unique challenges is an important consideration when aiming to generate knowledge to guide EBP within the context of child welfare. For example, much of the knowledge to guide EBP is generated in environments such as, residential settings, therapeutic clinical settings, or private practice with non-mandated clients. These settings are more stable and offer more opportunities for control than the child welfare environment offers. There are few other environments in which it is a new world everyday. Historically, a big focus of social work has been on context; the environment in which organisms exist, and process, the manners in which organisms do what they do. Thus, it is important that we incorporate these concepts in efforts to generate and evaluate evidence-based knowledge.

Study Limitations

This study was ambitious in that it aimed to explore the unexplored area of child welfare supervisory mentoring in a non-traditional manner. Although the final findings are expected to present information that will be valuable to the study participants and their agencies, for several reasons, project researchers must proceed carefully in projecting the findings across populations. The study used a sample of convenience, meaning no randomization was used in the assignment of workers to the experimental group or control group. This limitation will affect the ability to later draw generalizations about what the data reveals. In fact, to this point, no distinction has been made between the participant group and the control groups. Those distinctions will be made later in the process.

CONCLUSION

Respect and appreciation for basing one's practice on interventions that are scientifically tied to a proven outcome is warranted. While an important focus, a focus solely on the outcomes of an effort does not represent the breadth and depth that we have long embraced in social work. Such a limitation minimizes the capacity of scientifically-generated knowledge to be maximally helpful to EBP. For EB knowledge to be most helpful research must be conducted in such a way that it tells the whole story; a task which numbers alone cannot accomplish.

REFERENCES

Bandura, A. (1977). *Social learning theory*. Englewood Cliffs, NJ: Prentice-Hall.

Bernotavicz, F. D., & Bartley, D. (1996). *A competency model for child welfare supervisors*. Portland, OR: The Dougy Center.

Ellett, A., & Ellett, C. (2002). *Measures and Items for The Fall 2002 Survey of Professional Child Welfare Staff in The Georgia Division of Family and Children Services* (University of Georgia, School of Social Work).

Gleeson, J. P. (1992, Fall). How do child welfare caseworkers learn? *Adult Education Quarterly, 43*(1), 15-29.

Gleeson, J. P. & Philbin, C. M. (1996). Preparing caseworkers for practice in kinship foster care: The supervisor's dilemma. *Clinical Supervisor, 14*(1), 19-34.

Hayward, R. (2004). Informing health choices: Reflections of knowledge integration strategies for electronic health records. In A. R. Roberts & K. Yeager (Eds.), *Evidence-Based Practice Manual: Research and Outcome Measures in Health and Human Services* (pp. 29-45). New York: Oxford University Press.

Hornby Zeller Associates. (2005). *Arkansas mentoring supervisors project demographic and background characteristics of project participants*. Unpublished manuscript.

Kadushin, A. (1976). *Supervision in social work*. New York: Columbia University Press.

Kadushin, A. (1992). *Supervision in social work (3rd Ed.)*. New York: Columbia University Press.

Kane, D. (1991). *Strategies and dilemmas in child welfare supervision: A case study*. Doctoral Dissertation. City University of New York, NY.

McClintock, C. (2004). Integrating program evaluation and organization development. In A. R. Roberts & K. Yeager (Eds.), *Evidence-Based Practice Manual: Research and Outcome Measures in Health and Human Services* (pp. 592-597). New York: Oxford University Press.

McNeece, A. C., & Thyer, B. A. (2004). Evidence-based practice and social work. *Journal of Evidence-Based Social Work, 1*(1), 7-25.

McNeece, A. (2004). The seven secrets of a successful veteran evaluator. In A. R. Roberts & K. Yeager (Eds.), *Evidence-based practice manual: Research and outcome measures in health and human services* (pp. 592-597). New York: Oxford University Press.

Munson, C. (2002). *Handbook of clinical social work supervision*, (3rd edition). New York: Hayworth Press.

National Science Foundation. (1997). *User-friendly handbook for mixed method evaluations* (Frechtling, J., Sharp, L., & Eds.). Retrieved 10/31/2004, from http://www.nsf.gov/cgi-bin/getpub?nsf 97153.

Pecora, P. J., Whittaker, J. K., Maluccio, A. N., Barth, R. P., & with Plotnick, R. D. (1992). *The child welfare challenge: Policy, practice, and research.* New York: Aldine De Gruyter.

Roberts, A. R., & Yeager, K. (2004). Systematic reviews of evidence-based studies and practice-based research: How to search for, develop, and use them. In A. R. Roberts & K. Yeager (Eds.), *Evidence-based practice manual: Research and outcome measures in health and human services* (pp. 3-14). New York: Oxford University Press.

Rosen, A. (2003, December). Evidence-based social work practice: Challenges and promise. *Social Work Research, 27*(4), 197-208.

Rosenthal, R. N. (2004). Overview of evidence-based practice. In A. R. Roberts & K. Yeager (Eds.), *Evidence-based practice manual: Research and outcome measures in health and human services* (pp. 20-28). New York: Oxford University Press.

Shulman, L. (1993). *Interactional supervision.* Washington, DC: National Association of Social Workers.

Southern Regional Quality Improvement Center (2001). *Summary of the Results of the Needs Assessment.* University of Kentucky, College of Social Work.

Usher, C. L. (2004). Measuring and evaluating effectiveness of services for families and children. In A. R. Roberts & K. Yeager (Eds.), *Evidence-based practice manual: Research and outcome measures in health and human services* (pp. 423-429). New York: Oxford University Press.

Williams, A. B. (1997). On parallel process in social work supervision. *Clinical Social Work Journal, 25*(4): 425-435.

Yeager. (2004). Program evaluation: This is rocket science. In A. R. Roberts & K. Yeager (Eds.), *Evidence-based practice manual: Research and outcome measures in health and human services* (pp. 647-653). New York: Oxford University Press.

Zunz, S. J. (1995). The view from behind the desk Child welfare managers and their roles. *Administration in Social Work, 19*(2), 63-80.

doi:10.1300/J394v04n03_06

The Role of Supervisors in Developing Clinical Decision-Making Skills in Child Protective Services (CPS)

Jenny L. Jones, PhD
Gregory Washington, PhD
Susan Steppe, MSSW

SUMMARY. Due to the often chaotic and overwhelmed work environment of most CPS units in the state of Tennessee, staff are concerned that critical decisions made throughout the life of any given case are made quickly, with scant information, and with little time given to thoughtful analysis of information that is known. Since the eyes and ears of the frontline case manager are the primary tools in gathering case information, and given that many case managers may have only a few months of experience, we posed the question "how can specific supervisory behaviors better support the work of staff in the field, helping to educate case managers and improve their basic skills of interviewing and observation?"

The purpose of this article is to examine the applicability of clinical decision-making as a tool for effective skills building in child protective

---

Jenny L. Jones and Gregory Washington are affiliated with University of Tennessee, College of Social Work.

Susan Steppe is affiliated with The University of Tennessee, College of Social Work, Office of Research and Public Service.

[Haworth co-indexing entry note]: "The Role of Supervisors in Developing Clinical Decision-Making Skills in Child Protective Services (CPS)." Jones, Jenny L., Gregory Washington, and Susan Steppe. Co-published simultaneously in the *Journal of Evidence-Based Social Work* (The Haworth Press, Inc.) Vol. 4, No. 3/4, 2007, pp. 103-116; and: *Developing an Empirically Based Practice Inititative: A Case Study in CPS Supervision* (ed: Jenny L. Jones, and Paul Sundet) The Haworth Press, 2007, pp. 103-116. Single or multiple copies of this article are available for a fee from The Haworth Document Delivery Service [1-800-HAWORTH, 9:00 a.m. - 5:00 p.m. (EST). E-mail address: docdelivery@haworthpress.com].

Available online at http://jebsw.haworthpress.com

doi:10.1300/J394v04n03_07

services supervision. Based on a training intervention methodology designed to teach child protective services supervisors 'best practices' approaches as it relates to evidence based practice, and the opportunity for these skills to be modeled for first line workers, the article presents process data from the specifically designed learning lab (clinical decision-making), feedback from supervisors and middle managers regarding implementation (challenges and solution), and a review of the individual learning plans to assess the front line supervisors attitude regarding clinical decision-making. doi:10.1300/J394v04n03_07 *[Article copies available for a fee from The Haworth Document Delivery Service: 1-800-HAWORTH. E-mail address: <docdelivery@haworthpress.com> Website: <http://www.HaworthPress.com>*

KEYWORDS. Child welfare, evidence based practice, supervision, clinical decision-making

INTRODUCTION

The Southern Regional Quality Improvement Center (SRQIC) engaged four southeastern states in a project designed to improve the practice of child protective services (CPS) through strengthening and supporting the role of the frontline supervisor. With current trends to develop evidence based practice this project has focused on testing specific learning lab modules and supervisory support strategies that could lead to specify desired outcomes for staff. A major focus of the Tennessee project has been improving CPS performance in the area of clinical decision-making. The Tennessee Department of Children's Services (DCS) Administrative staff identified this particular focus as a key concern in several recent cases. The state of Tennessee is currently under consent decree due to a class action lawsuit brought on in 2000 by Children's Rights (a New York-based national advocacy group), on behalf of children in DCS' custody. As a result of the lawsuit, the Department began a re-structuring process that included a more streamlined and systematic approach to decision-making in child protective services. This approach called for a focus on 'best practices' that strive to bring services more in line with the best available clinical science with the goal of promoting those practices that have been demonstrated effective. The need for 'best practices' that are responsible, science based with stated outcomes are increasingly needed in child welfare agencies for a means of accountability and improved client measures (Rosen, 2003).

Research has demonstrated that decisions regarding child safety vary significantly from caseworker to case worker, even among those considered to be child welfare experts (Ellett, 2001). Inappropriate decisions can be costly, leading to an overuse and sometime abuse of out-of-home placements, or tragedy resulting in the injury or death of a child. Due to the often chaotic and overwhelmed work environment of most CPS units in the state, staff are concerned that critical decisions made throughout the life of any given case are made quickly, with scant information, and with little time given to thoughtful analysis of information that is known. Since the eyes and ears of the frontline case manager are the primary tools in gathering case information, and given that many case managers may have only a few months of experience, we posed the question "how can specific supervisory behaviors better support the work of staff in the field, helping to educate case managers and improve their basic skills of interviewing and observation?" Improvements in these areas were believed to be linked to improved decision-making, thus improving outcomes for children and job performance/satisfaction for staff.

In response to glaring inconsistencies in the decision-making process and ineffective practice, the Tennessee Supervisors' Development Project developed and implemented a series of specific learning labs. Clinical Decision Making-Parts I & II were one of six learning labs proposed as a part of the original program design (Jones, Alexander, & Patterson 2004). This lab focused on the usefulness of clinical decision making as an effective tool for supervisors. All labs were didactic in structure, equipped to provide supervisors with knowledge, competence, and confidence required to make critical decisions revelent to 'best practice approaches' in CPS. The labs included skill development activities, review of response priorities, planning for case closure, and mock staffings. The labs were followed with a series of mentoring sessions with supervisors to reinforce the concepts presented in the labs, and ways to implement concepts in the field. Seasoned professionals who attended the learning labs along with the supervisors conducted the mentoring sessions.

The purpose of this article is to examine the applicability of clinical decision-making as a tool for effective skills building in child protective services supervision. Based on a training intervention methodology designed to teach child protective services supervisors 'best practices' approaches as it relates to evidence based practice, and the opportunity for these skills to be modeled for first line workers, the article presents process data from the specifically designed learning lab (clinical decision-making), feedback from supervisors and middle managers regarding implementation (challenges and solution), and a review of the individual learning plans to assess the front line supervisors attitude regarding clinical decision-making.

DEFINING CLINICAL DECISION-MAKING

In order to establish a framework for clinical decision-making the project turned to the work of Dr. John Clark (University of Kentucky College of Social Work). Dr. Clark advocates the use of scientifically researched or "evidence based practice" (EBP) approaches to decision-making in child welfare and recognizes the barriers to making use of EBP in the course of a typical workday in the world of Child Protective Services supervisors and workers. Dr. Clark's assertion is supported and shared by other researches in the field (Gambrill, 1999; Gonzales, Ringeisen, & Chambers, 2002; Proctor & Rosen, 2004), who identify challenges both extrinsic and intrinsic that are inherent in the application of day-to-day practice that include decision-making based on evidence to support their effectiveness in attaining desired outcomes. The practice of evidence based consists of three components: practice wisdom formalized as "best practices" approaches (Clark, 2004); scientific evidence (Clark, 2004; Rosen, 2002), as recognized in peer-reviewed publications and presentations; and, a privilege of conclusions based on evidence rather than "guesses" or "hunches" (Clark, 2004). Proctor and Rosen, in press; Rosen, 2002, further suggest that practice should be regularly monitored with appropriate revisions based on outcome evaluation. All of these components require a huge commitment on the part of the supervisor. The need for this type of practice in child welfare has become more critical, particularly during times when child welfare agencies around the country are trying to provide effective interventions and proclaim efforts of best practice as a means for achieving specified outcomes. And yet, child welfare supervisors often encounter barriers that impede their ability to engage in such practice.

Factors Influencing Clinical Decision-Making

Research indicates that there are certain factors that influence clinical decision-making based on EPB approaches, and the process involves several elements: obstacles related to scientific findings, heuristics (mental short cuts) (Moody, 2005), accuracy, and organizational (Clark, 2004). Clark further asserts that each of these factors equally impacts the worker's ability to make a sound clinical-decision, whether it is in a team process or individually. Furthermore, it is noted that one fundamental challenge to practitioners' use of EPB approaches is there acceptance of pre-tested, standardized, empirically unsupported treatments as a legitimate foundation for practice. For example, Carrillo, Packard, and Clap (2003) reported results from a statewide study that included seventeen family support programs that most programs did not use their agency's information system to make case decision, despite the provision of training and technical assistance. Unfortunately, this lack of acceptance appears to be the norm in public child welfare. The obstacles stated above will be discussed in detailed and an example of there applicability will be described.

Scientific Findings

As widely acknowledge, obstacles to scientific finding are based on theoretical assumptions that all learning is *memory based*; decision-making relies on memory; cognitive structures are used to perceive the unstructured world; the use of mental short-cuts (heuristics) (Clark, 2004). In a case example:

> A supervisor is assigned a specific directive from the regional headquarters and time is of the essence. A newly assigned case manger walks in and interrupts with questions regarding "next steps" on a case that she was out late on yesterday afternoon. As the case manager begins presenting the issues surrounding the case, the supervisor moves quickly to think and act.

Because of time constraints and deadlines the supervisor's response relies on her experiences of other cases that "sound like this one." The supervisor's decision-making asserts that the decision was made strictly on memory. When rushed and distracted, the possibility of cognitive error increases and mental shorts cuts multiply.

Heuristics

Heuristics (mental short cuts) are used to organize perceptions and process information; heuristics are evolutionary advantages that can lead to adaptive or maladaptive "biases" that create "cognitive strain" (Clark, 2004; Moody, 2005). When this process occurs it allows one to turn novel situations into familiar ones. When applied, these scientific findings place limits on the clinical decision-making process and impacts the worker's ability to make a sound decision. Using the example stated above, the supervisor maybe thinking, "I do not have time to spend on this–I'm sure this case is just like all of the others," thereby avoiding "cognitive strain" and fitting this case into her common understanding (which might be erroneous) of all other cases that sound sort of like this one. Here, the supervisor moves quickly to make a decision about how the case should be handled. What may have been helpful, if the supervisor had scheduled a specific time later that day to meet with the worker and not feel pressured to solve the matter at that moment, may have been a way to model effective problem analysis and decision-making.

Accuracy

When discussing the use of accuracy or lack thereof as a factor when implementing EBP approaches, it is critical to understand that not all evidence is created equal; therefore it is not always accurate. Frost (2002) suggests that we should strike a balance which evidence is pursued in the real world and its limitations. Clark (2004) suggests that certain types of evidence, although important for some aspects of practice may be inadequate for determining effectiveness, therefore impacting the decision-making process. For example, anecdotal narratives about client outcomes may be a poor indicator of effective practice decision.

Obstacles to accuracy have a major impact on EBP approaches. Accuracy is classified into two dimensions: satisficing–and fear of uncertainty, error. Both dimensions play crucial roles in the decision-making process. *Satisficing, a form of accuracy and evidence* (when used improperly) is used to fight fatigue or lack of clarity, and allows the worker to come to closure very quickly, even if more data or deliberation is needed. *Fear of uncertainty, error*, manages "cognitive strain" and emotional reactivity (anger, fear) by using untestable, dichotomous approaches that favor security over accuracy. When these approaches are used the worker and supervisor will have a tendency to error on the side of best practices and use "gut" level instincts, which often prove fatal for the families.

Organizational Obstacles

Organizational obstacles encompass two approaches to clinical decision-making: groupthink and the Abilene effect. *Groupthink* involves the worker relying solely on the expressed opinions of the group to validate conclusions and decisions. This approach leads to poor decision-making, not to mention the potential harm it may have on the family. The use of groupthink alone to make a clinical decision is impractical and erodes the whole process of evidence-based practice. The *Abilene effect* refers to the worker relying on their ideas of what the group thinks or expects. Again, this approach limits clinical decision-making and leaves room for error to supercede sound judgment and effective practice.

As noted, each obstacle has a significant impact on EBP approaches used in clinical decision-making, whether in a team format or an individual process. The intended purpose of clinical decision-making as a part of evidence-based practice approaches is to improve the processes and outcome of service efforts and interventions.

Evidence Based Practice Component

The literature suggests that the availability of scientifically generated literature is a prerequisite to a child-welfare supervisor's ability to engage in EBP (Rosenthal, 2004). Moreover, the use of EBP practices has emerged as a predominant theme in the social work literature (Howard, McMillen, & Pollio, 2003; Moore, 2005). Professional organizations such as the Council on Social Work Education and the National Association of Social Work (NASW) support the basic principles associated with EBP (Proctor & Rosen, 2004). The Social Work Code of Ethics adopted by NASW indicates that practitioners have an obligation to use research-based inquiry to guide their professional decisions. And, as child welfare agencies around the country continue to remain under federal mandates that support the recruitment and hiring of professionally trained social worker the use of EBP becomes more crucial.

In contrast to the push from agency administrators for more accountable and science based practice, often times this approach is stymied and the various obstacles discussed above become the dominant mode of practice. In an attempt to address some of these obstacles, the Project engaged middle managers and supervisors in this analysis. This next section of the paper present results from a two-part learning lab that focused on supervisors and middle managers contextualization of the information presented on EBP and clinical decision-making.

SUPERVISORS AND MIDDLE MANAGER'S VIEWPOINTS ON CLINICAL-DECISION MAKING

A total of 29 supervisors and ten middle managers attended the two-part learning lab held over a 3-month period. The lab was a structured over a 1-1/2 day period for each part, held during the months of

March and June 2004. The labs were videotaped and all of the participants voluntarily agree to the sessions being videotaped. The stated purpose of the clinical decision module was to develop a common language among CPS staff regarding decision-making practices and present a framework for using this form of practice, while moving toward helping the Department accomplish its objective of improving CPS performance in the area of clinical decision-making.

A qualitative research approach that included focus groups was utilized to examine the feasibility of an evidence based clinical decision-making process. Participants were asked to pair into five groups and to develop top ten lists of reasons why the clinical decision-making model presented could work in their respective offices, and a top ten list of potential barriers as to why it would not work. After small group discussions were completed, it was agreed that the lists would be collapsed into two-master lists.

During part-II of the lab the results of the master lists were presented for discussion and feedback among supervisors and middle managers. Both agreed the master lists were reflective of the list of *reasons for* and list of *barriers*. The small group and larger group discussion appeared reflective of the styles and atmosphere that influence the process in which clinical decisions based on EPB approaches are made in the various CPS field offices. It is important to note that there was a fair amount of pessimism and frustration that surfaced throughout the discussion, which appeared to be a reaction to experiences of resistive or indifferent responses to proposed change. Feedback from some supervisors indicated a theme of "We have already tried some of this," that is comparable to one of the "Big Three" Heuristics (anchoring) where the practitioner stay's with their first impressions and is not interested in moving away from it (Clark, 2004). This mindset undergirds the varying perspectives throughout the literature related to the lack of implementation of EBP approaches.

The facilitated discussion related to the identified theme allowed the opportunity for the various approaches to be conceptualized and influenced the outcomes of the lists of *reasons* for and *barriers*. The process of developing these lists contributed to understanding the perceived barriers of the organizational practices, policy, and culture. It also clarified the commitment and willingness to change that was expressed by many of the participants. However, there appeared be consensus among the group that EBP approaches are important to decision-making, therefore important enough to try and implement. Table 1 identifies the specific reasons for and barriers to implementing EBP approaches in clinical

TABLE 1. Master list of *reasons for* and *barriers to* implementing clinical decision-making

Top Ten Reasons It Could Work	Top Ten Barriers	Obstacles Related EBP
1. Evidence Based = Accuracy	1. Workload (Caseloads/paperwork)	1. Mental short-cuts
2. Credibility to decision making team	2. Lack resources	2. Satisficing
3. Asking more questions is okay	3. Time (Lack of Timeframes)	3. Mental short-cuts; memory based
4. Incorporates additional variables	4. Lack of skill set	4. Memory-based & Mental short-cuts
5. Improve errors that contribute to learning	5. Policy/Procedures (Task driven, inconsistencies)	5. Satisficing/ groupthink
6. Contributes to flexibility (Open-mindedness)	6. Punitive nature of Dept. (Errors are bad)	6. Mental short-cuts; memory-based
7. Promotes knowledge building (Staff development)	7. Inflexible leadership	7 Organizational
8. Contributes to creativity	8. Turnover	8. Organizational
9. Encourages hypothesis testing	9. Legal complexities (Judges, GALS & CPS vs. Staff)	9. Mental short-cuts, Memory-based, & Satisficing
10. Awareness of biases is valuable	10. Organizational Culture (Resistant to change)	10. Groupthink / Albeline effect

decision-making, as defined by the supervisors and middle managers. In addition, an example of the appropriate obstacle(s) related to EBP that supports the barrier is also referenced.

The combined lists in their separate functions indicate that clinical decision-making, utilizing EPB approaches is important to child welfare practice, but before it can be adopted a number of extraneous variables (organizational issues) must be addressed. These lists were also analyzed through process research methodology (content analysis) and the following themes were identified:

1. an agreed upon understanding of clinical decision-making
2. level of practice (EPB) is related to accuracy

3. organizational constraints, i.e., policies and procedures, leadership and poor resources.

The initial two themes reflect supervisors and middle managers support for EBP approaches as a component to clinical decision-making. The third theme is reflective of many of the extraneous variables (i.e., organizational issues) that some supervisors and managers believed that were beyond their control. Moreover, the final theme appears to be more extrinsic in nature, in that the supervisors and middle managers voiced their inability and lack of power to make fundamental change in their respective field offices. Supervisors and middle mangers consistently agreed that while they believed they could have some impact on integrating clinical decision-making however, change related to the barriers as they relate to organizational constraints included in the top ten list was limited. Overall, both supervisors and middle managers linked "organizational constraints" to their administrative duties particularly when it referred to the rapid policy changes, lack of resources (e.g., high caseloads, not enough staff, instability in senior level management), and insurmountable paperwork within the organization. Kadushin 1992 notes this function of supervision as a frequently cited concern when it comes to the role of the supervisor. These commonly cited reasons are consistent with the literature related to the current state of public child welfare agencies around the country (London & Smither, 1995; Fleenor & Prince, 1997).

How Can the Individual Learning Plan (ILP) Assist in the Development of Clinical Decision-Making Skills?

The development and implementation of the clinical decision-making module using components of EPB would be meaningless without feedback, evaluation, and development of a plan of action from the participants. Therefore, the Individual Learning Plan [ILP] (see Appendix) was used as a tool by the supervisors to identify goals and objectives, and specific tasks they would be willing to implement in their respective offices in an effort to build on the classroom learning. The ILP is a critical aspect of this process, in that it allows for behavioral and organizational change to be documented.

Approximately 4-weeks following the 2-part learning labs, supervisors met with respective mentors to further discuss and develop learning plans. The plans outlined specific tasks and skills to be completed over the next three months regarding EBP and clinical decision-making. A supervisor/mentor signed copy of each ILP was filed with the research team. Content analysis of *learning plans* reflected the following:

- "I will schedule and adhere to weekly case conferences with each case manager on my team. These meeting will allow for discussion of each case and provide direction to the case manager."
- "I will work to model effective problem-solving techniques with my team by selecting one case per month and complete a case staffing."
- "I will begin with staying committed to the already scheduled weekly case conferences with my team."

Follow-up with supervisors by assigned mentors to track the progress of the stated individual learning plans took place via face-to face, telephone, and/or email contacts. At the conclusion of Year-2 of the project (Summer 2004) most of the supervisors had completed a partial plan. As the project moved into its third and final year of the intervention (Fall 2004), attrition became a concern as the number of supervisors had significantly decreased (through resignation, re-assignment, and promotions) to 18 versus the 29 who participated in the 2-part learning lab. As the project moves into the final phase of the intervention component (Spring 2005), an individual review with each supervisor of the stated goal will be recorded. Subsequently, an item comparison analysis linking the stated goal with the outcome of the clinical training will be conducted.

LESSONS LEARNED

Over the course of the 2-1/2 year collaborative partnership between Tennessee's public child welfare organization, state university social work program, and community partners, numerous lessons have been learned. First, the spirit of "true collaboration" is critical to the success of any project of this kind. The Tennessee project, from the beginning has been met with a combination of challenges beginning with selection process, to implementation of the intervention, to the constant changes in administration at the state level. These confounding variables have impacted significantly every aspect of the project. Second, professional growth and development is essential for supervisors and middle managers in order for them to remain competent and stay abreast of current trends in child welfare. When supervisors have the opportunity to engage in self-directed growth, they often are empowered to improve their own behavioral functioning and model this behavior for their workers. Third, the use of EBP components in clinical decision–making should involve a systematic method for evaluating how supervisors perform their role, and requires the support of administration. Fourth, supervisors understanding of evidence based or 'best practices' was greatly enhanced as indicated on their individual learning plans, which alone may reduce internal conflict when faced with complex decisions and a limited amount of time to make them. Finally, organizational constraints are among the confounding variables that must be addressed in order to integrate EBP components into clinical decision-making. Supervisors regularly reported during mentoring sessions and at scheduled trainings their levels of frustration over continuous policy changes from central office and the impact these changes have had on their ability to implement this particular learning lab, as well as the other labs presented over the 2-year period in the manner that they would have like to.

While the outcome of clinical decision-making skills among supervisors in the various field offices is inconclusive at this time, the experience supports the contention that specifically targeted behaviors can change when the appropriate tools (the ILP) are used as a mechanism for feedback and assessment. A critique of the literature related to clinical decision-making, and the use of content analysis to identify themes from the process data indicate that a balanced approach to clinical supervision overall increases supervisors ability to be empowered to improve their approach to decision making, as well as role model this behavior for their workers (Gibbs, 2001). While this 2-part learning lab and the use of the ILP can be documented as useful tools for making an impact on changing worker practice and organizational culture in public child welfare agencies, support of and commitment to appropriate resources is crucial if the organization is to realize its potential for service improvement.

REFERENCES

Carrillo, T.E., Packard, T., & Clapp, J.D. (2003). Nothing in–nothing out: Barriers to the use of performance data in social service programs. *Administration in Social Work, 27*(4), 61-76.

Clark, Jim (2004, March). *Clinical Decision Making.* Invited presentation at the Tennessee Supervisors Development Project Training, Nashville Tennessee.

Ellett, A.J. (2001). *Child welfare self-efficacy beliefs in two states: Implications for employee retention and practice.* Paper presented at the Society for Social Work and Research 5th Annual Conference, Atlanta, GA.

Fleenor, J., & Prince, J. (1997). *Using 360-degree Feedback in Organizations: An Annotated Bibligraphy*. Greensboro, NC: Center for Creative Leadership.

Frost, N. (2002). A problematic relationship? Evidence and practice in the work place. *Social Work and Social Sciences Review, 10*(1), 38-50.

Gambrill, E. (1999). Evidence-based practice: An alternative to authority-based practice. *Families in Society, 80*, 234-259.

Gibbs, J.A. (2001). Maintaining front-line workers in Child Protection: A case for refocusing supervision. *Child Abuse and Review, 10*, 323-335.

Gonzales, J.J., Ringeisen, H.L., & Chambers, D.A. (2002). The tangled and thorny path of science to practice: Tensions in interpretering and applying "evidence." *Clinical Psychology: Science and Practice, 9*(2), 204-209.

Howard, M.O., McMillen, C.J., & Pollio, D.E. (2003). Teaching evidence-based practice: Toward a new paradigm for social work education. *Research in Social Work Practice, 13*, 234-259.

Jones, J.L., Alexander, D., Patterson, N. (2003). Tennessee Supervisors Development Project. *Journal of Professional Development*, (6)1/2, 74-78.

Kadushin, A. (1992). *Supervision in Social Work (3rd edition)*. New York: Columbia University Press. London, M., Smithers, J. & Adsit, D. (1997). Accountability" The Achilles' heel of multisource feedback. *Group and Organization Management,* 22:2, 162-184.

Moody, J. (2005). *Rising Above Cognitive Errors: Guidelines for Search, Tenure, and other Evaluation Committees* [www.DiversityOnCampus.com].

Moore, B.C. (2005). Empirically Supported family and peer interventions for dual disorders. *Research on Social Work Practice, 15*(4), 231-245.

Proctor, E. & Rosen, A. (2005). Concise standards for developing EBP guidelines. In Roberts, A.R., & Yeager, K.R. (Eds.), *Evidence-Based Practice Manual: Research and Outcome Measures in Health and Human Services*, (pp. 193-199). New York: Oxford University Press, Inc.

Roenthal, R.N. (2004). Overview of evidence-based practice. In .Roberts, A.R. & Yeager, K.R. (Eds.), *Evidence-Based Practice Manual: Research and Outcome Measures in Health and Human Services*, (pp. 193-199). New York: Oxford University Press, Inc.

Rosen, A. (2002). *Evidence-based social work practice: Challenges and promise*. Invited address at the Society for Social Work and Research, San Diego, CA.

Walker, R. & Clark, J. (1999). Heading off boundary problems: Clinical supervision as a risk management. *Psychiatric Services, 50*(11), 1435-1439.

doi:10.1300/J394v04n03_07

APPENDIX

INDIVIDUAL LEARNING PLAN

Name:____________________ Supervisor: ________________

Length of time in current role :______________________________

Date of plan:____/____/____

1. Competency to be developed:

2. How would you rate the current level of proficiency?

3. Description of the level of proficiency you hope to achieve:

4. Learning activities you will use:

Activity	Who will help
A.	
B.	
C.	
D.	

5. What is you plan for following up this learning plan? List concrete steps and the dates when they will be completed:

1. Date:____/____/____

2. Date:____/____/____

3. Date:____/____/____

Systematic Case Review Data and Child Protective Services Outcomes: The Development of a Model in Mississippi

Kimberly K. Shackelford
Maxine Harper
Kathleen Sullivan
Tiffany Edwards

SUMMARY. Child welfare agencies have recognized the need for accountability and the value of using data for decision-making. However, there are few indicators that child welfare supervisors are using outcome data to make decisions affecting the performance of child welfare workers and/or client outcomes. Child welfare supervisors who are participating in the Mississippi QIC learning labs are using case review data summaries to compare outcomes for project evaluation purposes and to facilitate changes in supervisory practices. The supervisors' review of case review data and their discussion of the meaning of these data enable and encourage supervisors to use data driven supervisory techniques to improve outcomes. doi:10.1300/J394v04n03_08 *[Article copies available for a fee from The Haworth Document Delivery Service: 1-800-HAWORTH. E-mail address: <docdelivery@haworthpress.com> Website: <http://www.HaworthPress.com> © 2007 by The Haworth Press, Inc. All rights reserved.]*

Kimberly K. Shackelford, Maxine Harper, Kathleen Sullivan, and Tiffany Edwards are all affiliated with the University of Mississippi.

[Haworth co-indexing entry note]: "Systematic Case Review Data and Child Protective Services Outcomes: The Development of a Model in Mississippi." Shackelford, Kimberly K. et al. Co-published simultaneously in the *Journal of Evidence-Based Social Work* (The Haworth Press, Inc.) Vol. 4, No. 3/4, 2007, pp. 117-131; and: *Developing an Empirically Based Practice Inititative: A Case Study in CPS Supervision* (ed: Jenny L. Jones, and Paul Sundet) The Haworth Press, 2007, pp. 117-131. Single or multiple copies of this article are available for a fee from The Haworth Document Delivery Service [1-800-HAWORTH, 9:00 a.m. - 5:00 p.m. (EST). E-mail address: docdelivery@haworthpress.com].

Available online at http://jebsw.haworthpress.com

doi:10.1300/J394v04n03_08

KEYWORDS. Child protective services, child welfare system, measurable outcomes, organizational culture, social worker self-efficacy, strengths-based perspective

INTRODUCTION

In the 1993 *Creating a Government that Works Better and Costs Less: Report of the National Performance Review,* Vice President Al Gore wrote "the federal government is not simply broke; it is broken." (Shafritz & Ott, 2001, p. 460). Gore (1993) also stated that federal programs appear to be designed to not work and perhaps are not designed at all. Sims (1998) discussed The National Performance Review of 1993, noting that President Clinton called for the creation of learning organizations instead of organizations only concerned with survival and legitimacy. Sims reported that the Government Performance and Results Act of 1993 called for performance plans to be a part of budgets submitted by agencies to the congress. Government agencies were to include a mission statement, goals and objectives that included outcomes and how these outcomes were to be achieved. Sims stated public agencies are under pressure to be accountable. "Agencies will have to run differently, jobs must be redefined, and learning and change need to be incorporated (and institutionalized) throughout the organization" (Sims, 1998, p. 1).

Child welfare agencies have been brought under public scrutiny along with other governmental agencies. Barth and Jonson-Reid (2000) stated demands for accountability and the pressure to determine outcomes regarding child welfare services may be greater now than they have been in the past. Courtney, Needell and Wulczyn (2004) discussed the federal government's attempts "to hold states accountable for achieving quantifiable outcomes for children involved in the child welfare system" (p. 1142). The Adoption and Safe Families Act of 1997, P. L. No. 105-89 Section 203(a) required the Secretary of the Department of Health and Human Services working with state public officials responsible for child welfare programs (governors, legislators and local administrators) to develop measurable outcomes and a system of rating performance with respect to the outcome measures and to then report the findings annually to the Congress. Measurable outcomes were determined for state child welfare agencies, and in March 2000 the Child and Family Services State Reviews were established. These put in place a mechanism for assessment of state child welfare systems in the areas of safety, permanency and wellbeing of children and families (Courtney et al., 2004). At the turn of the century, as state child welfare agencies faced mandates calling for new governmental performance ratings and measuring outcomes, as well as public demands for accountability, the agencies were also implementing new automated information systems. State Automated Child Welfare Information Systems (SACWIS) were funded in part by the federal government through the Omnibus Budget Reconciliation Act of 1993 (P. L. 103-66) (Courtney, Needell, & Wulczyn, 2004). The Title IV-E Social Security Act (1986) had already required the establishment of the Adoptions and Foster Care analysis and Reporting System (AFCARS) and then the SACWIS requirements were translated into requirements for the National Child Abuse and Neglect Data System (English, Brandford, & Coghlan, 2000). English et al., claimed that child welfare was quickly increasing the development of administrative databases but that the development and use of the databases presented administrators with challenges along with opportunities. For these data systems to be useful, the administrative data must be integrated into policy development, practice innovations, and the development of program outcomes (English et al., 2000).

DATA USE IN CHILD WELFARE

Schoech, Quinn, and Rycraft (2000) claimed that even though the child welfare information systems were growing in sophistication, few child welfare agencies used the data for decision-making. Schoech et al., quoted Naisbitt (1982) and agreed that employees were often drowning in data, but are starved for knowledge. Data mining was determined by Schoech et al. to be a new field for child welfare. Because of the tremendous amount of data made available from the new information systems, frontline social workers and administrators need new skills to "sift through voluminous data and records to extract knowledge for decision-making" (Schoech et al., 2000, p. 633). Although the possibilities for data mining are greater with new information systems being developed, English, Brandford, and Coghlan (2000) claimed that there were two determining factors regarding the actual usefulness of data in the development of child welfare policy and practice. Usefulness is determined by the following questions: (1) Are the data reliable? (2) Are the data integrated into the decision-making process? The answers to these questions must both be affirmative in order for the data to have "long-term viability" (English et al., 2000, p. 450). Even if the data are reliable (which requires accurate and complete data input), English et al. claimed that data-based organizational change would not occur if no one values or uses the information.

Data-based organizational change will not occur if the data are not used however, organizational change is necessary for the data to be used in child welfare agencies. Schoech, Quinn, and Rycraft (2000) discussed data mining in child welfare and stated that a new managerial task for administrators is to design systems by which employees have access to collective knowledge and have training to use the knowledge to improve job performance. Schoech et al. called the collective knowledge "organizational intelligence." In order for an agency to have "intelligence," everyone in the organization is responsible for collecting, entering, and using the data (Schoech et al.). Schoech et al. claimed that intelligent organizations are created when employees share, learn and improve through the use of data and worker expertise. "Knowledge management involves systematically capturing organizational information and expertise, integrating it, and making it interactively available to employees who are trained to use it in decision-making to achieve goals" (Schoech et al., 2000, p. 634). Schoech et al. also concluded that creating organizational intelligence requires cultural change. The change would involve the inclusion of workers in organizational knowledge building, with everyone involved being responsible for complete and accurate data (Schoech et al., 2000).

Even when the data are complete and accurate, very often the amount of data is too much for child welfare social workers and administrators to handle. When it becomes overwhelming, employees may find it easier to ignore the data than make sense out of the volumes of information (Jamieson & Bodonyi, 1999). Jamieson and Bodonyi claimed that data gathered by child welfare agencies should be relevant to the goals of child welfare and "should be used to instigate, direct, and monitor change efforts" (p. 16). Jamieson and Bodonyi researched the Families for Kids program in Washington State as project personnel used data to develop new policies and to measure change (Jamieson & Bodonyi). Jamieson and Bodonyi reported that social workers, supervisors and top policymakers involved in the Families for Kids project used the data to develop solutions in the field, rather than as a punitive tool. The researchers on this project also discussed "data-brokering" as the managerial act of sifting and filtering for useful data.

Researchers working with the Families for Kids project also found that sometimes the data were difficult to hear and accept and the tendency of workers was to try to discount the data. Jamieson and Bodonyi (1999) reported that when workers vocalized disbelief about the credibility of the findings, the local workers were then responsible for examination of data collection and data entry. The social workers and supervisors in the field were not passive recipients of negative data but instead were given frameworks in which to formulate solutions that fit their clients in the environment in which they worked (Jamieson & Bodonyi). Authors of the study noted that the workers were given direction and allowed to explore further issues and that work was done to prevent hopelessness when data revealed situations which needed enormous improvement. The project showed that system change occurs when there is an integration of data, policy, and fieldwork. Jamieson and Bodonyi concluded that data are powerful and useful to workers when the data are relevant to stated goals and when data are meaningful and simple.

Usher, Wildfire and Gibbs (1999) attributed the reluctance to use data to measure performance of child welfare agencies to fear that data would add to the ammunition of persons wanting to measure the negative rather than the positive work done by child welfare workers. Agency workers fear this would worsen the public's pessimistic attitude toward child welfare agencies. After reviewing findings from evaluations of reform initiatives in Alabama, North Carolina, and Ohio, Usher et al. stated that performance systems "must be adaptable to changing circumstances, particularly when improvements in one area can affect standards and expectations in others" (Usher, Wildfire, & Gibbs, 1999, p. 1).

Even though the use of data to measure outcomes has been shown to be essential for child welfare professionals to move toward improved performance and better outcomes for children and families, Moore, Rapp, and Roberts (2000) reported little evidence that outcome data were being used by field supervisors in the field of child welfare. After a three year project in Kansas that focused on developing the capacity of child welfare managers to use data to improve performance, Moore, Rapp, and Roberts suggested that three conditions must be present if managers are to use data. The reports must be easy to read and use, the organizational culture must be supportive of learning and outcome achievement, and managers must know how to use the data to achieve desired outcomes.

Mississippi's Southern Regional Quality Improvement Center Project

Mississippi's Southern Regional Quality Improvement Center project incorporated these conditions into the design of a series of learning labs for child welfare supervisors. In an effort to create learning environments which use data to support changes in practice that can possibly improve outcomes for clients, the Mississippi Child Protective Services Casework Supervision Demonstration Project has used a case review system designed by the Mississippi Department of Human Services–Division of Family and Children's Services. The report generated from this case review system had been received by the supervisors prior to participation in the learning labs. Prior to participation in the learning labs, the report was not being used by the social workers, supervisors or middle managers. Supervisors said they did not consider case review data to be valuable because (1) an enormous amount of data appeared in each report and it was hard to read, (2) the data showed very few cases reviewed as having satisfactory work in any area under review, (3) the reviewer's standards were not viewed as the same as the supervisor's standards for approving social worker's work, and (4) the situation was too overwhelming to begin to make efforts to correct the problems (especially with high caseloads, worker vacancies and worker turnover).

One objective of the Mississippi SR QIC is to create regional Learning Laboratories that will provide collaborative problem-solving, program evaluation and practice improvement that build lasting competence in public and private agencies throughout the region's protective services. The child welfare supervisors have focused on evidence-based practice improvements, measurement of outcomes and improvement of child welfare delivery systems. The child welfare supervisors participating in the learning labs found that instead of not using the case review system it would be better to work towards making the case review system beneficial to them.

HISTORY OF THE DEVELOPMENT OF CASE REVIEW DATA IN MISSISSIPPI

The Children's Bureau within the U.S. Department of Health and Human Services has developed outcome-based standards for assessing quality in child protective services. In applying these standards through Child and Family Services Reviews conducted over a three-year period, the Children's Bureau found that no state was in full compliance with federal standards (Pear, 2004). The Bureau's review process focused attention on the federal government's intention to hold states accountable for meeting specific outcome-based standards in child welfare.

Some states have adopted the federal government's outcome-based model in developing their own standards for assessing services for in-home child welfare cases. Unlike criteria for traditional case reviews, which focus on compliance with agency casework policies, outcome-based case reviews are used to measure the extent to which agencies achieve specific safety and well-being outcomes.

The Mississippi Department of Human Services–Division of Family and Children's Services developed an outcome-based case review system that began statewide (seven of nine regions) use in 2003. The Mississippi Case Review included collection of data consistent with data gathered by federal reviewers through Child and Family Services Reviews, as well as additional data beyond that required by federal guidelines. The Department of Human Services developed a data base for compiling and summarizing case review data from the seven participating regions.

QIC Project Use of Case Review System for Evaluation of Project

The QIC project researchers along with supervisors and managers from the child welfare agency chose indicators from the data available in the Mississippi Department of Human Services case review system that could be affected by improvement in clinical casework supervision. Project evaluators analyze quarterly data on the selected indicators to assess changes in case outcomes in participating regions. The case review has many more indicators than the items included in the evaluation of this project. Table 1 presents a comparison of the content of Mississippi's system for assessing in-home case outcomes which have been used by project evaluators and the indicators use by federal reviewers in the CFSR system.

The evaluation design of the project is quasi-experimental as two regions with 10 supervisors each were chosen to be the intervention group and two regions with 10 supervisors each were chosen to be the control group. Data from each region are being compared to identify differences in outcomes that might be associated with improvements in supervision in QIC regions. The evaluation results are not included at the time of this writing as only preliminary data has been collected. The project is a three year project and the last data will be collected during Fall 2005. The project is attempting to create a cultural shift regarding the use of data in decision-making and even the end-of-project data can only be considered preliminary. The mid-project measures have been used for formative evaluation purposes and have helped in refining project implementation.

TABLE 1. Child Protective Service Outcomes and Case Review Data Collected for each Outcome–Indicators used in the Mississippi QIC project

Outcome	Data Collected through Mississippi's Case Review System which coincides with federal CFSR	Additional Data Collected by Mississippi beyond That Required by the Federal Child and Family Services Review
Safety Outcome 1: Children are, first and foremost, protected from abuse and neglect.		
Item 1: Timeliness of initiating response to a child maltreatment report	• Assigned within 24 hours of report date • Initiated within 24 hours of report date • Face-to-face contact with victim within time frame	• Primary Abuse/Neglect • Reports considered satisfactory for region review of who was contacted during investigation and if proper supervisory reviews were done to determine if considered to be done at a satisfactory level–standards met–yes or no • For each type of interview during investigation a review is done to determine if the interview was done satisfactory (victim, parent(s)/caretaker(s), perpetrator, other household members)
Item 2: Repeat Maltreatment	• Number of repeat maltreatment in which evidence was found • Number of repeat maltreatment in which same perpetrator was found • Number of reports in which same general maltreatment was found	• Safety plans considered satisfactory
Safety Outcome 2: Children are safely maintained in their homes whenever possible and appropriate.		

Item 3: Services to family to protect child(ren) in home and prevent removal	
Item 4: Risk of Harm to children	• number of primary assessments considered satisfactory • number of assessments in which risk, safety and well-being are consistent with initial assessment and investigation findings • collecting data regarding individual service plans • number of adult isp's considered satisfactory • number of goal statements considered satisfactory • number of assigned tasks considered satisfactory • number of corresponding achievement criteria considered satisfactory
Well-being Outcome 1: Families have enhanced capacity to provide for their children's needs.	
Item 19: Worker Visits with Child(ren)	• Average number of monthly successful face-to-face contacts between child(ren) and social worker • Number of monthly face-to-face contacts between child & worker that appeared to have a definitive purpose or objective
Item 20: Worker Visits with Parent	• with family preservation services and without for each of the following number of monthly successful face-to-face contacts • mother–social worker • father-social worker

TABLE 1 (continued)

Outcome	Data Collected through Mississippi's Case Review System which coincides with federal CFSR	Additional Data Collected by Mississippi beyond That Required by the Federal Child and Family Services Review
Well-being Outcome 2: Children receive appropriate services to meet their educational needs.		
Item 21: Educational Needs of Child	• Number of identified educational issues that are not being addressed, but need to be addressed.	
Well-being Outcome 3: Children receive adequate services to meet their physical and mental health needs.		
Item 22: Physical Health of the child	• Number of identified medical issues that are not being addressed, but need to be addressed • Number of identified dental issues that are not being addressed, but need to be addressed	
Item 23: Mental Health of the child	• Number of identified mental health issues that are not being addressed, but need to be addressed	

Although Mississippi's case review process was implemented in 2003, Mississippi lost several social worker positions due to state budget cuts and therefore in 2004, Mississippi discontinued its systematic case review process in the seven regions of the state in which it had been implemented. The reason given was that the case reviewers were needed to work in the field doing investigations or working with clients. In response to a request by Mississippi's QIC project personnel, the Department of Human Services agreed to continue conducting reviews on an abbreviated basis in the four regions involved in the QIC project to enable continued evaluation of the project and for other uses in the project. The case reviews previously had been conducted on all in-home cases opened during a specified quarter. Although three case reviewers returned to field work as a result of personnel cuts and staff shortages, one reviewer continues to review a random sample of in-home cases opened during the specified quarter.

Mississippi's SR QIC evaluators use regional case review data summaries to measure the effectiveness of the QIC Learning Lab intervention. Outcomes of the two regions with Learning Labs have been compared with those of two regions without Learning Labs to identify differences in performance on case review standards for three quarters in fiscal year 2004. Evaluators used these data to determine which regions had the highest percentage of items on which standards were met. In addition, evaluators were able to track progress of regions in meeting standards across the quarters for which data were collected. This use of systematic case review data demonstrates the utility of outcome data for evaluating the effectiveness of various interventions that may be implemented in an effort to improve supervisory practices and service provision at the county and regional levels.

In addition to the use of outcome data in the SR QIC project evaluation, case review data also are central to the Learning Lab intervention. Through supervisors' review of outcome-based case review data and discussion of the usefulness of these data, supervisors are encouraged to improve outcomes using case review data. The following describes the value of this type of data to supervisors and the learning process involved in the use of data to promote better practice.

The SR QIC Learning Lab Intervention and Its Use of Outcome Data

The key element of the SR QIC model is the Learning Lab. Area Social Work Supervisors from two regions (10 counties each) participate in

Learning Labs offered in each region. A unique element of this model is that the supervisors determine the topics to be discussed in the Learning Labs through a participatory democratic process. As topics arise in the lab, research and planning is done for future labs to incorporate new area of interest and to consider needed knowledge and skills.

The goal of this process is to achieve buy-in from the supervisors and to allow for topics that are relevant and useful to the supervisors. The topics focus on improvement of clinical casework supervision in the child welfare agency. The labs are a mixture of information from research, skill development and discussion of ethics and values. Attitudes, beliefs and feelings are also discussed. The supervisors offer true case scenarios from their own supervisory units for the application of theory and practice skills as well as the application of problem solving and decision making processes. The Learning Labs also have resulted in the development of supervisory tools that can be shared with other child welfare supervisors after the supervisors have piloted them in their own units. Participants have determined that future Learning Lab group members also need to participate in the development of tools, as the process has been as important as the finished product.

The design of the model includes the use of the participatory democracy to encourage sharing of work and information among supervisors between the times of the Learning Labs. One of the elements of the model is to encourage the use of research in child welfare practice by field supervisors and social workers. The intervention groups have begun to include articles and book chapters on empirically based practice and supervisory skills in regular supervisory staff meetings. Supervisors give input and bring information that they have read to staff meetings and Learning Labs. Another element of the program is to encourage the supervisors and social workers to be life-long learners with the goal of continual improvement of practice. The supervisors in turn use the Learning Lab model with social work staff. This element of the model is important in promoting the continuation of empirically based practice among all staff members after the demonstration project ends.

Use of data to improve practice is also an important element of the project. Supervisors have delved into data generated from MACWIS (Mississippi Automated Child Welfare Information System) reports and the Case Review System reports. The process of reviewing the reports has not been easy and many struggles have ensued during the learning labs. The first struggle involved the overwhelming amount of data the supervisors have placed in their hands. The tendency was to let the reports pile up on their desk or they were filed without being read.

Allowing the supervisors time to read the reports in the learning labs has led to the supervisors being able to determine what data helps and what data is not helpful in the reports. The next hurdle was to sift through the data to determine if the data input was correct. This has identified data input issues that have been discussed with social work staff.

Supervisors then struggled with assessments and case plans being determined unsatisfactory by the reviewer when the supervisor had approved these parts of the case record. Much discussion continues regarding this issue as practice among supervisors and social workers has been determined to be inconsistent at times and regarding different issues. Policy is being interpreted in slightly different ways which leads to some degree of inconsistent practice. The documentation in the case record does not always allow for a reviewer to know what has occurred with the client. Assessments have been found to not always include every issue which needs to be addressed and case plans have been found to need improvement. The work of the social workers is good but the supervisors are learning by digging into the data that there is room for improvement in the documentation and in some areas practice. This is not surprising to the supervisors given the results of the Child and Family Service Review but it is sometimes a surprise that some of the problems exist in the area under their own supervision. The supervisors were quick to think that the problems were in other supervisors' areas.

The discussion regarding data uses a strengths-based perspective. Supervisors and middle managers examine data from the counties that are doing well on various outcomes and discuss what that region is doing that allows for better outcomes. Participants also discuss what the data really show and what other data need to be collected and analyzed to present a better picture of what is really happening with clients.

Teambuilding is a crucial element of the Learning Labs. The Learning Labs have improved working relationships among supervisors. Purposeful teambuilding has allowed a high level of trust among the members of each group that has resulted in honest sharing of needs and thoughts in the labs. The trust, genuineness and belief that the supervisors need to help each other have allowed for risk-taking in the sharing of new ideas and also with the sharing of supervisors' feelings about the difficult issues that arise in the field of child welfare. Resource sharing has occurred between counties and supervisors and is beginning to occur between the two intervention regions as a result of this effort.

CONCLUSIONS

In reviewing the literature related to use of data in child welfare agencies, data mining to filter large volumes of data and records to extract knowledge for decision-making has become an effective method to facilitate organizational change. One change needed relates to data. Data needs to be valued and then used in the determination of practice and policy. Despite the fact that child welfare professionals' use of data to measure outcomes has been demonstrated to be essential in moving toward improved performance and better outcomes for children and families, there is little evidence that outcome data are being used by child welfare supervisors.

The Children's Bureau within the U.S. Department of Health and Human Services reviewed states to determine their compliance with outcome based standards in child welfare and found that no state was in full compliance with federal standards (Pear, 2004). To address the deficiencies in use of outcome data to promote best practices and high standards being met in the field of child welfare, the Mississippi project of the SR QIC has designed a series of Learning Labs for child welfare supervisors. These labs use regional case review data summaries to promote changes in supervisory practices that have the potential for improving client outcomes. Comparisons between regions that used Learning Labs (intervention regions) and regions that did not use these labs (control regions) are serving to help evaluators determine if differences exist in performance on case review standards between the intervention and control regions. The data is preliminary, especially when considering the complex and deeply-rooted problems faced by the child welfare system. Further, the systematic case review data has allowed evaluators to track progress of regions in meeting standards. The use of systematic case review data appears to be showing that outcome data can be useful for evaluating the effectiveness of given interventions on the improvement of supervisory practices and service provision at the county and regional levels. In addition, supervisors' review of outcome based case review data and their discussion of the meaning of these data enable and encourage supervisors to use data driven supervisory techniques to improve outcomes. One other result of supervisors digging into reports and data has been a review of data input for accuracy.

The child welfare supervisors, as participants in the learning labs, have discussed a progression of use of data within the child welfare agency. The discussion has revealed a change from looking at "is work being done?" to looking at "what are we doing?" The supervisors stated that the cases have been reviewed for compliance (Is there a case plan in the record?) but they want to know if the work being done is good work or best practice (Is the case plan appropriate and on target regarding the work to be done with the client?). The case reviews currently attempt to ask the questions regarding appropriateness and adequacy of the work being done. The next question to be asked will be "Is the work being done effective?" Are families and children better off for having been involved with the child welfare agency?

REFERENCES

Adoption and Safe Families Act of 1997. P. L. No. 105-89.

Barth, R. P., & Jonson-Rein, M. (2000). Outcomes after child welfare services: Implications for the design of performance measures. *Children and Youth Services Review, 22*(9), 763-787.

Courtney, M. E., Needell, B., & Wulczyn, F. (2004). Unintended consequences of the push for accountability: The case of national child welfare performance standards. *Children and Youth Services Review 26*(12), 1141-1154.

English, D. J., Brandford, C. C., & Coghlan, L. (2000). Data-based organizational change: The use of administrative data to improve child welfare programs and policy. *Child Welfare 79*(5), 499-516.

Gore, A. (1993). Creating a government that works better & costs less: Report of the national performance review. In Shafritz, J. M., & Ott, J. S. (Eds.) (pp. 460-468). *Classics of organization theory*. Belmont, CA: Wadsworth Group/Thompson Learning.

Jamieson, M., & Bodonyi, J. M. (1999). Data-driven child welfare policy and practice in the next century. *Child Welfare 78*(1), 15-31.

Mission of the Quality Improvement Centers. (n.d.). Retrieved January 11, 2005, from http://www.uky.edu/SocialWork/trc/indexqic.html.

Moore, T. D., Rapp, C. A., & Roberts, B. (2000). Improving Child Welfare performance through supervisory use of client outcome data. *Child Welfare 79*(5), 475-498.

Pear, R. (2004, April 26). U.S. finds fault in all 50 states' child welfare programs. *The New York Times*. Retrieved January 7, 2005, from http://www.nytimes.com/2004/04/26/politics/26CHIL.html

Schoech, D., Quinn, A., & Rycraft, J. R. (2000). Data mining in child welfare. *Child Welfare 79*(5), 633-651.

Sims, R. R. (1998). *Accountability and radical change in public organizations*. Westport, CN: Quorum Books.

Usher, C. L., Wildfire, J. B., & Gibbs, D. A. (1999). Measuring performance in child welfare: Secondary effects of success. *Child Welfare 78*(1), 31-52.

doi:10.1300/J394v04n03_08

Longitudinal Research Design and the Realities of Changing Practice Environments: The Difficulty in Testing Models for Evidence Based Practice– A Case Study

Susan C. Steppe, MSSW
Jenny L. Jones, PhD

SUMMARY. The primary goal of the Tennessee demonstration project was to strengthen and expand a coordinated approach to casework supervision of frontline CPS caseworkers by developing and implementing a series of comprehensive, culturally sensitive learning labs modules that will increase the effectiveness of frontline supervision and improve client outcomes (Jones, Alexander, & Patterson, 2004). This paper focuses on the external variables that impacted the development and implementation of the Tennessee Project. It further offers strategies that may be useful in addressing these variables. doi:10.1300/J394v04n03_09 *[Article copies available for a fee from The Haworth Document Delivery Service: 1-800-HAWORTH. E-mail address: <docdelivery@haworthpress.com>*

Susan C. Steppe is affiliated with University of Tennessee Knoxville, College of Social Work, Office of Research and Public Service.

Jenny L. Jones is affiliated with University of Tennessee Knoxville, College of Social Work Nashville Campus.

[Haworth co-indexing entry note]: "Longitudinal Research Design and the Realities of Changing Practice Environments: The Difficulty in Testing Models for Evidence Based Practice–A Case Study." Steppe, Susan C., and Jenny L. Jones. Co-published simultaneously in the *Journal of Evidence-Based Social Work* (The Haworth Press, Inc.) Vol. 4, No. 3/4, 2007, pp. 133-143; and: *Developing an Empirically Based Practice Inititative: A Case Study in CPS Supervision* (ed: Jenny L. Jones, and Paul Sundet) The Haworth Press, 2007, pp. 133-143. Single or multiple copies of this article are available for a fee from The Haworth Document Delivery Service [1-800-HAWORTH, 9:00 a.m. - 5:00 p.m. (EST). E-mail address: docdelivery@haworthpress.com].

Available online at http://jebsw.haworthpress.com

doi:10.1300/J394v04n03_09

KEYWORDS. Public child welfare, evidence-based practice

INTRODUCTION

The Southern Regional Quality Improvement Center (SRQIC) engaged four Southeastern states in a project designed to improve the practice of child protective services (CPS) through strengthening and supporting the role of the supervisor. The primary goal of the Tennessee demonstration project was to strengthen and expand a coordinated approach to casework supervision of frontline CPS caseworkers by developing and implementing a series of comprehensive, culturally sensitive learning labs modules that will increase the effectiveness of frontline supervision and improve client outcomes (Jones, Alexander, & Patterson, 2004). Specifically, the project is a collaborative endeavor that includes Tennessee's public child welfare agency (Department of Children Services-CPS Unit), the state's public university (University of Tennessee College of Social Work), and community partner, (the Tennessee Citizens Review Panelist). It was noted in the SRQIC's request for application, this level of collaboration allows for an approach to service delivery that will better serve populations that may not be reached in a more traditional service delivery model.

This paper focuses on the external variables that impacted the development and implementation of the Tennessee Project. It further offers strategies that may be useful in addressing these variables.

TENNESSEE'S DEVELOPMENT PROJECT

The conceptual framework for the overall design of the project was based on Schulman's theory (parallel process) that focuses on quality and structure of interaction between the worker and supervisor–parallels that of the worker and the client (Schulman, 1993). The model is strength-based, promotes critical thinking, peer consultation, via case discussion and peer-group meetings, and on-site mentoring. The overall goal is to create an environment where transfer of knowledge and skills can take place and increased education, via clinical guidance imbued in a supportive relationship. The format for the model includes a series of learning labs, held in a classroom type environment conducted by experienced trainers (Jones, Alexander, & Patterson, 2004). The on-site technical assistance (mentoring component) was a critical feature of the overall design of the project in that it was used to reinforce the knowledge gained during each lab and allowed for hands on learning, including modeling, direct observation, and feedback through the use of actual case activity. Below is a brief description of each module:

Module I: Educative Supervision

Objective: To build on the educative supervision framework that encompasses adult learning theory, learning styles, and assess worker/supervisor needs for learning.

Module II: Ethics

Objective: To introduce ethical decision-making in clinical practice, which focuses on how values and ethics shape practice approaches, and supervisory techniques that enhance problem solving around ethical conflict.

Module III: Cultural Competency

Objective: To introduce a framework for working with cultural differences, whether it is other ethnic group, cultural groups, or other minority groups.

Module IV: Clinical Decision-Making and Evidenced-Based Practice

Objective: To use evidenced-based practice techniques (theory and research) demonstrated through individual and group supervision, case conferences, etc., with the goal of increasing the supervisor's clinical skills, and contribute to their practice knowledge, and increases analytical skills.

Mentorship

The process of mentoring was a major component of the overall delivery of the learning labs. Mentorship, defined as an interpersonal helping relationship between two individuals who are at different stages in their professional development (Collins, 1994). The mentoring process involves modeling and on the job training activities directed at training supervisors to become mentors to newly hired supervisors and current supervisors. This phase of the learning is designed to strengthen supervisor's knowledge and reduce stress among supervisors and caseworkers, reduce worker turnover, and increase overall effectiveness of job satisfaction, which will ultimately increases service delivery and outcomes to clients.

WHY ENGAGE IN A RESEARCH-BASED PROJECT?

A major focus of the Tennessee project has been related to improving CPS' performance in the area of clinical decision-making. In the often chaotic and overwhelmed work environment of most CPS units in the state, there is concern that critical decisions made throughout the life of any given case are made quickly, with scant information, and with little time given to thoughtful analysis of information that is known (S. Abernathy, personal communication, September 6, 2002). The eyes and ears of the frontline case manager are the primary tools in gathering case information, and given that many case managers may have only a few months of experience (DCS, Human Resources Report, 2005), we posed the question, "how do specific supervisory techniques better support the work of staff in the field, helping to educate case managers and improve their basic skills of interviewing and observation." Improvements in these areas were believed to be linked to improved decision-making, thus improving job performance (Diwan, Berger, & Ivy, 1996), job satisfaction (Newsome & Pillari, 1991; Rouktis & Koeske, 1994), and turnover in staff (Ellett & Millar, 2001; Schoen et al., 2001; Cicero-Reese & Black, 1998; Harrison, 1995; Whelly & Miracle, 1994). The interventions implemented toward development of these goals included a series of learning labs as outlined above. Seasoned professionals who served as mentors attended the same training sessions as those attended by the supervisors conducted the mentoring sessions. The research effort was designed to explore the relationship between these training activities and subsequent outcomes including turnover rate for CPS case managers and improved job satisfaction for supervisors.

THE CHALLENGES IN PUBLIC CHILD WELFARE

The SRIQ's efforts to conduct a project using scientific research designs in the public child welfare sector represents a bold step in defining "best practice" in the area of public child welfare services. According to findings of the Kaufmann Best Practices Project (2004), it has only been in recent decades that the mental health treatment community, which relied on anecdotal information from experienced practitioners for many years, has sought to develop empirically based interventions to benefit victims of child abuse and neglect. Given that the mental health treatment profession, which is more accustomed to constructing and implementing research efforts, has been slow to move into this arena, it is not surprising that there are few examples longitudinal research efforts in the public child welfare arena. A review of the child welfare literature indicates that few empirical studies have focused on supervision in general; the use of best practices techniques remain understudied in public child welfare. Tsui conducted a review of supervision research in 1995 and found only 30 empirical articles on supervision over the last 30 years. Most of these studies documented functions of supervision with attempting to evaluate effectiveness.

Daily Process in CPS

From the outset, the field of child protective services provides a chaotic background to attempt to structure and implement scientific research designs. The number of reports and size of caseloads is a central problem in child protection (United States General Accounting Office, March 2003). CPS staff are mandated to respond to all reports that are considered appropriate for investigation and have little ability to pace themselves or control workload size. Additionally, the cases themselves are emotionally charged, involving families struggling with numerous, serious problems, or families who are less problematic, but angry about having been the subject of a report. Either way, in most instances families are not happy to see a CPS caseworker standing at the door; emotions run high in these interactions.

Others factors such as, fear of inappropriately identifying the presence of abuse or neglect, possible media attention, and the remote chance of legal action for personal liability, and the stress of this work environment are compounded. In addition to these challenges that are inherent to child protection, the Tennessee project staffs faced numerous other hurdles in the organizational culture that influenced implementing the research design. These issues are discussed below.

ORGANIZATIONAL CHANGE

Changes in Leadership

Changes in program leadership within the Department have had a significant impact on the implementation process of this project; affecting the degree of ownership or lack of ownership exhibited by key central office leadership of the TDCS. The original proposal and project was constructed and "sold" by the Director of Child Protective Services who clearly supported and believed in the project. Yet, the director was obligating the Department to participate in the effort while at the same time preparing to retire from the agency. That support for this effort certainly helped in the agency's agreement to "sign on" to the project, but the retirement of the director left the implementation phase in the hands of the university partners, with no assigned person in a leadership role from within the department available to nurture the program in its early stages. This change coupled with subsequent changes in leadership at the Commissioner's level left the project in something of a "no man's land"–a swell idea that no one really wanted to own, but felt they could not abandon since the CPS unit could obviously benefit from additional support and training.

The lack of enthusiastic support at the core management level was transmitted to or sensed by the intervention group, which affected their attitude toward participation. Overwhelmed participants were already skeptical about the benefits of this program. When they sensed ambivalence in the top ranks of management they grew more skeptical and their resistance to participate increased. This resistance became a major factor in the implementation of the project.

Shifts in Organizational Priorities

The frequent changes at the Commissioner and Program levels of the organization affected the priorities for frontline staff and further contributed to general feelings of instability and unpredictability in the work environment. Each new leader took time to survey the new territory, re-arrange the organizational chart, and establish a new set of priorities. The most recent leadership has focused on two key aspects of child protection–response time and timeliness of completion of investigations. Improved data collection has made it possible to produce reports that specify worker and unit performance on these two issues. Thus these issues are currently a driving force in child protective services practice in Tennessee. While these issues are not incompatible with a desire to improve decision-making, there has not been an effort to connect these priorities to the concepts of sound clinical decision-making, due in part to the management changes mentioned above. Conceivably, one could respond to a report and complete an investigation in a timely manner and yet, fail to make a sound decision. In the absence of a clear connection between organizational priorities and the concepts of clinical decision-making, the project has been perceived as more remote or "not applicable" to the present work environment, further fueling participant resistance.

Impact of Random Selection

While regions were randomly selected for participation, supervisors were allowed to make a choice as to whether or not to participate. After the regions where chosen for participation there was communication with each Regional Administrator from the selected regions, and each agreed to participate, voicing support for the project. After Regional Administrators agreed to participate, each supervisor was informed that this was a voluntary endeavor and they had the opportunity to opt out of participating if he/she desired to do so. While this certainly sounds like an opportunity for free choice, is it really? Given that Central Office had ordained the project and Regional leadership had approved it, it is not reasonable to expect individual supervisors to refuse to participate? This moment illustrates a major challenge in conducting this type of project in the public agency environment. Large agencies of this nature employ a "chain of command" philosophy, and there may not be a great deal of tolerance for those who attempt to operate outside of that structure. Even when participants were given the opportunity to opt out of the program, they may have believed that they would experience negative consequences for refusal. Once again this "offer you cannot refuse" relates to participants' attitudes and perceptions of the project and their ability to embrace the experience as a valuable opportunity.

Selection of Mentors

A critical aspect of this project was the provision of one-on-one mentoring to each supervisor. Theoretically, after each training module was delivered, the mentors would meet with the participants to reinforce understanding of the concepts and discuss ways to implement these concepts in the field environment. They would offer support and the opportunity to brainstorm solutions to the real world problems. In this scenario, the relationship between the mentors and the supervisor participants is critical to the success of this venture. Given the nature of this work, the mentors should have been carefully selected for their skills and knowledge in child protection issues, in the functioning of child welfare organizations, and in the development of professional supportive relationships.

Unfortunately, the selection process did not meet these criteria for several mentors. Because of the need to put the project in place within a short timeframe (another product of organizational change), several professional staff persons from the central office CPS program unit were assigned the task of "mentor" as an addition job task. Once again freedom of individual choice emerged as a critical issue. These persons were not truly interested in performing the mentoring role. Furthermore, some stated that they were ill prepared to play a mentoring role to the frontline supervisors; a concern that was also expressed by the supervisor participants. This process for selection of some mentors compounded negative feelings about the project, led to mentor "turnover," and certainly impacted the ability to develop the very relationships that were believed to be essential to achieving desired outcomes in the project.

High Profile Cases

In the course of this project the Tennessee Child Protective Services program was the subject of much media attention due to perceived problems in the performance of duties on the part of some staff. There were at least 4 high profile cases that involved seriously injured children who had a prior history with the Department. In response to these cases several staff persons were subject to the disciplinary process and some staff subsequently left the Department's employment. While there is no way to measure the impact of these events on the implementation of the project, there is much anecdotal information to suggest that these cases with the concomitant media attention and personnel actions have had a great impact on staff attitudes and perceptions toward their jobs. It appears that these events have weighed heavily on the minds of the CPS staff and are believed to have contributed to less job satisfaction and more staff turnover, the very outcomes, which the project was seeking to influence and improve.

Lawsuits

Throughout the course of the project the State of Tennessee has been striving to comply with settlement agreements stemming from several law suits. Specifically, the Brian A lawsuit was the most pressing, in that DCS was obligated to make substainual change in its operating procedures. While child protective services was not the central focus for this suit or any of the suits, the many complex activities that are required to aspire for full compliance limited the amount of time and resources that can be devoted to the child protective services program.

IMPLICATIONS FOR PRACTICE

While there is no way to control for all of the possible changes and external variables that can affect the operation of a longitudinal study, the following concepts may prove useful as lessons learned from the Tennessee experience.

Identifying Advocates or Sponsors

It is critically important that some group of individuals is totally committed and willing to serve as "spark plugs" and spokespersons for a project of this nature. There must be at least one central office staff person who has the ability to access the highest leadership. Additionally, it is critical to win or co-opt key program leaders in the field who recognize the long range benefits from the project and are willing to voice this to others. There should be a back-up plan or alternate assigned for each of these persons, planning ahead for departures or transfers. These plans should be written and approved by every level of leadership.

Develop a Strong, Concise Message

Any research effort that requires child welfare staff to attend additional meetings and filling out computerized questionnaires can seem far removed from the frantic demands of their work. It is important to develop a strong, one-page message that concisely conveys what the project is, why we are doing this, what we hope to accomplish, and why this is important to the field of child welfare. This document should be drafted in partnership with all concerned partners for use by the advocates mentioned above as well as with external partners in the community when speaking about and support of the project in the field.

Efforts to Engage Participants

The Tennessee project could have offset some of the resistance to participation in the project from the onset through allowing participant input into the development of the project, giving participants the opportunity to identify training topics and helping to define the scope and nature of the mentoring experience. While is it important to establish adequate parameters to maintain the integrity of the research design, some latitude in this area is essential in overcoming the strong influence of an initially unwilling participant group who perceives that their participation is mandatory.

It's critical to allow staff the opportunity to voice their concerns about project participation. Hearing these issues early in the process and trying to address participants' concerns to the greatest degree possible is essential to winning their confidence to continue with the project and to see it as an opportunity where one can speak freely.

Another critical factor include providing secondary rewards for participants. This proved to be a positive aspect of the project. The chosen meeting locations allowed for participants to be more relaxed and engaged in the process. These locations were aesthetically pleasant and appealing for training sessions, and they allowed for lunch to be catered. These small types of incentives convey a positive message to staff that rarely receive small perks. This may also help to create a sense of pride in project participation.

Identify and Respond to Concerns Early On

The project staff must be ready and willing to hear concerns of participants when they are first expressed. Ignoring a participant's dissatisfaction or failing to respond to stated concerns only contributes to the belief that participants are truly trapped into the project.

It is evident that the variables indicated in this paper had a great impact on the overall success of the project. While the discussion related to each variable is based on the Tennessee experience, it is likely that these concerns are echoed in public child welfare around the country.

CONCLUSION

Any effort to implement a longitudinal research design in the public child welfare sector must combat the critical issues described here. The backdrop of constant organizational change, revolving priorities, and struggling staff morale interferes with efforts to construct and implement a research effort that allows for randomly selected participants, crisply defined and well-operationalized variables, fidelity to the proposed intervention, and consistent data collection. Yet, the work to protect vulnerable children through effective intervention with their families is highly valued in our society. If we ever hope to establish evidence-based best practice guidelines for Child Protective Services, we must combat and overcome the obstacles that create and maintain the chaotic and unpredictable work environment.

REFERENCES

Cicero-Reese, B., Black, P. (1998). Research suggests why child welfare workers stay on the job. *Partnerships for Child Welfare, 5*(5), 8-9.

Diwan, S., Berger, C., & Ivy, C. (1996). Supervision and quality assurance in long-term care case management. *Journal of Case Management, 5*(2), 65-71.

Ellett, A., & Millar, K. (2001). *Child welfare self-efficacy beliefs in two states: Implications for employee retention practice*. Paper presented at Society for Social Work Research 5th Annual Conference, Atlanta, GA.

Harrison, S. G. (1995). *Exploration of factors related to intent to leave among child welfare caseworkers.* Doctoral dissertation, Ohio State University.

Jones, J. L., Alexander, D., Patterson, NM. (2004). Tennessee Supervisors Development Project. *Journal of Professional Development, 6*(1/2), 74-78.

Kauffman Foundation. (March 2004). Closing the Quality Chasm in Child Abuse Treatment: Identifying and Disseminating Best Practices. A collaboration of Chadwick Center for Children and Families of the Children's Hospital–San Diego, CA.

Newsome, M. Jr., Pillari, V. (1991). Job satisfaction and the worker-supervisor relationship. *The Clinical Supervisor, 9*(2), 119-129.

Schoen, S., Goodson, J., King, J., & Phillips, M. (2001). *An exploratory evaluation of former child welfare stipend students who are currently employed at DCFS in Arkansas*. University of Arkansas.

Schulman, L. (1993). *International supervision.* Washington, DC: National Association of Social Workers.

Tsui, M. (1997). The roots of social work supervision: A historical review. *Clinical Supervisor, 15*(2), 191-198.

United States General Accounting Office. (2003). *Child Welfare: HHS Could Play a greater role in helping child welfare recruit and retain staff.* (GAO Publication No. 03-357). Washington, DC: Author.

Whelly, J., & Miracle, H. (1994). Practicum Education: A practice partnership for family preservation. In *Empowering Families: Papers for the Seventeenth Annual Conference on Family Based Services.* Riverdale, IL, National Association of Family Based Services.

doi:10.1300/J394v04n03_09

Using 360 Degree Evaluation to Improve Clinical Skill Development by First Line Child Protective Services Supervisors

Michael J. Kelly, PhD
Paul Sundet, PhD

SUMMARY. Didactic skill training in clinical practice techniques is insufficient to assist first line child protective supervisors in the difficult task of changing a child welfare organization's culture to emphasize the therapeutic aspects of intervention. Supervisors need assistance in personal growth based on accurate feedback from performance. When such feedback is coupled with targeted individual development plans, evidence from a two year intervention demonstrates that significant behavioral changes do occur and these can be linked to organizational outcomes. doi:10.1300/J394v04n03_10 *[Article copies available for a fee from The Haworth Document Delivery Service: 1-800-HAWORTH. E-mail address: <docdelivery@haworthpress.com> Website: <http://www.HaworthPress.com> © 2007 by The Haworth Press, Inc. All rights reserved.]*

KEYWORDS. Public welfare, supervision, clinical skill, clinical training

---

Michael J. Kelly is affiliated with the School of Social Work, University of Missouri-Columbia.

Paul Sundet is affiliated with the School of Social Work, University of Missouri-Columbia.

[Haworth co-indexing entry note]: "Using 360 Degree Evaluation to Improve Clinical Skill Development by First Line Child Protective Services Supervisors." Kelly, Michael, and Paul Sundet. Co-published simultaneously in the *Journal of Evidence-Based Social Work* (The Haworth Press, Inc.) Vol. 4, No. 3/4, 2007, pp. 145-161; and: *Developing an Empirically Based Practice Inititative: A Case Study in CPS Supervision* (ed: Jenny L. Jones, and Paul Sundet) The Haworth Press, 2007, pp. 145-161. Single or multiple copies of this article are available for a fee from The Haworth Document Delivery Service [1-800-HAWORTH, 9:00 a.m. - 5:00 p.m. (EST). E-mail address: docdelivery@haworthpress.com].

Available online at http://jebsw.haworthpress.com

doi:10.1300/J394v04n03_10

INTRODUCTION

The principle role of any supervisor, to use the famous analogy of Rensis Likert (1961) is to be a linking pin that holds an organization together. Quality supervision is the keystone to quality service in organizations with relatively high turnover of first-line staff and where that staff come to the agency with limited professional education. And no where is this more important than in child protective services. With the multiple and competing demands of child protection, child well-being, parental rights and community interest continually pulling at workers and administrators alike, it falls to the child protective services supervisors to mediate, educate and model appropriate practice and to establish the mores governing day-to-day intervention with children and their families (Brohl, 2004; Wagner, van Reyk, & Spence, 2001; Shama, McKelvey, Hardy, Epstein, Lomax & Husby, 1997).

Much has been written about the need to change the culture in child welfare to make it both more responsive and more effective in performing its difficult societal functions (e.g., Lind, 2004; Hutson, 2004; Casey Family Services, 2003; Snell, 2000; Orr, 1999). Because the supervisors serve as "culture carriers," persons who set the practice and organizational atmosphere within which the caseworkers function, they carry a special burden in helping organization change (Kadushin, 1992). One of the authors (Kelly) has also explored the culture carrying role of the supervisor as expressed through mentoring (Kelly, 2001; Kelly & Lauderdale, 1999).

This article addresses the use of systematic evaluation and feedback on the performance of first line supervisors in a state child welfare agency. Based on a training intervention methodology designed to teach supervisors 'best practices' in clinical skill building and allow them to model these skills for the first-line worker, the study reports the results of using a 360 degree evaluation methodology, professional feedback and individual learning plan development to evaluate (1) changes in worker, peer and superior's assessment of the first-line supervisors in five skill/knowledge areas: (2) how structured feedback and individual development planning model the skill and knowledge building process and (3) how supervisors use clinical skill development with their workers.

Clinical Skill Building Within a Culture of Compliance

The Missouri Children's Division (CD) had, for some time, been seeking to find ways in which to better equip that agency's supervisors for this task and to refocus efforts to emphasize the clinical oversight rather than the surveillance aspects of their function. When completive Children's Bureau funding became available through the Southern Regional Quality Improvement Center for a three and one-half year demonstration, a coalition of the Division, the University of Missouri-Columbia School of Social Work (SSW), Prevent Child Abuse Missouri (PCAM) and Missouri Alliance for Children and Families (MAC-F) was formed to develop an intensive experimental staff development project designed to produce and measure changes in supervisor behavior and the impact of that change on safety and well-being of children in the caseloads they oversee. The approach chosen for emphasis was "role demonstration" in which the supervisor performs in actual or simulated environments the tasks and skills the workers are expected to learn (Mermelstein & Sundet, 1978). This model was adopted based on research with the workers that concluded they had sufficient traditional classroom type instruction but needed and wanted practical demonstration and mentoring in case-specific techniques from their immediate supervisors (Sundet, Mermelstein & Watt, 2003).

Because research of the effectiveness of the proposed model was a core component of the project, the participants were limited to supervisors in two administrative units, one an urban/metro area and the other a distinctly rural region. The total number of supervisors in the training group was 35. Passive comparison groups of like size were drawn from matched areas of the state. A multi-method approach was developed to evaluate changes in supervisory methods and the effect on case based outcomes. Among the measures (not reported in this study) were relative changes in Peer Record Reviews, consumer satisfaction, Federal child welfare outcomes, and preventable staff turnover. The authors also employed a cultural change evaluation based on the Survey of Organizational Excellence (Lauderdale, 1999) and two scales measuring worker self-efficacy and self-efficacy outcomes (Ellett, 2001). Changes in supervisory skills were also assessed by two qualitative methods–annual focus groups and instructors' evaluations provided. The complete evaluative plan can be seen in Bolm, Pettit, Kelly, and Wolchko, 2003.

EVIDENCE BASED ISSUE

While the philosophical and pedagogical conceptions of the project were clear from the onset, substantial time and effort were expended in defining precisely what would be the most appropriate staff development interventions to concentrate on. Division administration, the supervisors themselves and their workers were all engaged in this analysis. The list of needs and wants was long and varied. However, in addition to the clinical skills and techniques that were identified as needing emphasis, a pervading malaise was evident. Although on the whole a dedicated and mostly graduate trained cadre, these supervisors demonstrated many of the traits that other research has found to be prevalent among child welfare workers including burnout, alienation and manifest stress (Child Welfare League of America, 2003; Evans, Bryant, Owens & Kelly, 2004; Stevens & Higgins, 2002; Lloyd, King & Chenoweth, 2002).

And while there is no consistent body of research that points to a high correlation between job satisfaction and individual performance (Iaffaldano & Muchinsky, 1985; Brayfield & Crockett, 1955), there is consistent evidence that low job satisfaction results in the negative characteristics noted above (Barling, Wade & Fullagar, 1990; Brooke & Price, 1989). Consequently the challenge became one of discovering paths through which satisfaction could be increased.

Research on job satisfaction has most often focused on extrinsic components such as pay or promotional opportunities or on issues of job structure (Ting, 1996; U.S. Merit System Protection Board, 1990; Lewis, 1987; Daley, 1986). In the Missouri system, pay is certainly a consideration where child welfare supervisors starting salaries lag from two to ten thousand dollars a years behind the contiguous states (Sundet & Cowger, 2004; Child Welfare League of America, 2003). However, impacting that disparity was beyond the scope of this project. Likewise, enhancing promotional opportunities was limited by existing structure although, as the project progressed, participants were singled out for advancement. And contrary to research in industrial settings, in child welfare the nature of the work itself, although stressful, does not appear to be a significant source of dissatisfaction (Sundet & Cowger, 1990).

In contrast to the "extrinsic" approaches to satisfaction among professional staff there is ample empirical evidence to support other approaches to impacting job satisfaction. Historically, management theory has emphasized the importance of the potential for growth for enhancing employee performance and work satisfaction (Hackman & Oldham, 1976; Hackman & Lawler, 1971; Herzberg, 1968; Likert, 1967; McGregor, 1960; Maslow, 1954). Feedback and career development opportunities appear to have significant impact on professional employees' satisfaction ratings and productivity (Taylor, 1999). A related factor is the importance of performance appraisal fairness in affecting overall satisfaction (Blau, 1999; Organ, 1988; Daley, 1986). Formal feedback is the key to activating this process (Taylor, 1999). Related to this research are studies which have found that support for employees' development efforts is vital to promoting productive use of appraisal feedback (Emmert & Taher, 1992).

Consequently the challenge became one of finding means to engage the supervisor-trainees in a data-based developmental process that had both credibility with them and one in which their immediate managers and the entire management structure would actively participate. A number of alternatives were considered but the one finally agreed on coupled the technology of 360 performance assessment, professional feedback and a structured form of Individual Development Plan.

The 360-Degree (Full Circle) Evaluation

A 360 evaluation can and does take many forms both in the public and private sector and is variously referred to as multi-source or multi-rater assessments (Lepsinger & Lucia, 1997; U.S. Office of Personnel Management, 1997). In its simplest form it is designed to provide a full-circle overview of a person's performance on the job by soliciting feedback from superiors, peers, direct reports and self on behaviors that are specific to the job assignment (Waldman & Atwater, 1998). The intent is to allow each individual to understand how her/his effectiveness as a subordinate, co-worker or superior is viewed by others in the organization who have the most immediate daily interaction with that person. Individuals providing feedback are generally limited to those staff with whom the employee routinely interacts.

Multi-source feedback has been researched in a broad range of public and private setting for more than twenty-five years and has proven, with certain caveats, to have significant impact on performance development (Fleenor & Prince, 1997; London & Smither, 1995). Full-circle feedback from work associates is generally viewed as both more credible and more motivating to the participants than the traditional single rater model commonly found in human service agencies (Heathfield, 2001). Used as a springboard for professional growth, this form of assessment can make a powerful impact on an individual's career and overall organizational effectiveness (Warrick, 1992). Its utility can be attested to by the fact that almost half of the 750 major United States firms reviewed by the American Society for Training and Development now employ the technique (Sugrue, 2003).

Among the positives that are cited as reason to employ a 360 evaluation process are that it provides well-rounded feedback from a number of sources, increasing the validity and reliability of performance judgments (Hoffman, 1995; Kirksey, 1994). It promotes teamwork by helping members understand how they are perceived by peers and assists in making members more accountable to one another because of their shared input into each others performance (Leslie & Fleenor, 1998). The feedback received is a crucial way of understanding each employee's unique developmental needs by providing information on what he/she needs to do to enhance career (Kluger & DeNisi, 1996; Auteri, 1994). The feedback is more accurate and more validating than that from a superior alone and more likely to be acted upon. And finally, the 360 also serves as an organizational barometer, providing valuable insights into organizational climate and morale.

But the 360 process is not without its shortcoming and pitfalls (Coggburn, 1998; Haworth, 1998; Wimer & Nowack, 1998). In some (many) environments, it has been used as a substitute for the total performance management system and tied to completive compensation judgments. A second failure has been to not have the behaviors on which feedback is being given clearly tied to the performance expectations of the job. A lack of understanding of the process and insufficient training of the participants has caused problems in some organizations. And a level of professionalism is required throughout the system to ensure that rating do not become simply a means of ventilating frustration or, conversely, a mutual feel-good exercise with reference to the reality of practice (Atwater & Waldman, 1998; London, Smither & Adsit, 1997).

Ghorpade (2000) reviewed more than 600 feedback studies, principally from for-profit organizations, concluding that about one-third reported that performance was improved while another one-third reported decreases in performance and the remainder showed no impact on performance. Nevertheless, Pafu (2002) encourages the use of full-circle feedback provided that steps are taken to insure effective feedback. Among the admonitions are to use the feedback for the right purposes, such as development rather than final performance decisions, and training people, particularly superiors in giving feedback. It should be noted that many of the reported studies noted that full-circle feedback was given to the subject without any assistance in interpretation.

In the Missouri implementation both the positives and negatives were carefully weighed and plans made accordingly. First, a 360 format that had been successfully used with social service supervisory personnel in other settings was chosen (Organizational Excellence Group, 2000) and the participants were given detailed oral and written instructions on its use. Considerable time was allotted to answer questions and address unique structural arrangements.

Great pains were taken to ensure that the responses would be confidential. The form for rating was individually computer generated with unique identifier codes known only to the rater and the external data compiler. The results of the assessment were used for developmental purposes only with the results the property of the individual supervisor. In some instances the participants decided to share the information with their superiors as part of the agency's performance management process but it was clearly negotiated with and understood by upper management that the 360 process was not part of the Division's personnel evaluation process and that the data were controlled by the recipient of the rating.

An absolutely essential element in effectively using this technique was tying the assessment data to an Individual Development Plan (IDP). Project personnel from the SSW met individually with each supervisor for an extended debriefing and discussion of the rating results. Discussions centered on both performance strengths and areas identified for improvement. Each supervisor then drafted an IDP and submitted it to the project director for input and consultation. At the conclusion of that process the supervisor then met with her/his immediate manager for further refinement of the plan which was then signed off on by all parties. This IDP was then a roadmap for the supervisor's development activities during the following year and performance was jointly evaluated by the supervisor and project staff consultant at the period.

PROCESS AND FINDINGS

The findings reported here concern the first project year (PY1) and the second years of the three year intervention. The 360 evaluation instrument is composed of five sections with six questions in each section (total of 30 questions) which ask the rater to judge the subject on a scale ranging from strongly agree (5) to strongly disagree (1) with a "not applicable" option. The instrument measures reactions to the subject's performance as a communicator, leader, manager, facilitator and professional. Respondents can also enter open-end comments in each area and are asked for open-ended comments regarding the subjects' areas of strength, areas to improve, and general comments.

The 360 evaluation instrument was explained during one of the formal training sessions and a demonstration on how to access and complete the Web based survey was given. Methods for protecting anonymity of the respondents was discussed and every supervisor was provided with a packet with instructions for completing a self-evaluation and instructions for distribution on up to twenty (20) respondents. The packets contain coded personal identification numbers (PIN) which the supervisors are instructed to distribute in a manner which insures that they will not know and respondent's PIN, They are asked to select persons they report directly to (their superiors), other supervisors filling the same job responsibilities (peers) and individuals reporting to them (direct report workers). A two week window was allowed for the respondents to complete the assessments. Completed data was returned in 10 working days with each supervisor receiving a confidential report with the average response scores for all respondents as well as those for the superiors, peer and subordinate along with their self-evaluation. The standard deviation for respondents' scores is provided along with the scale average score from past administrations of the instrument.

Along with mean scores for each question, the report provides a bar graph of the five areas overall scores and a mean score for all five areas. In addition, bar graphs for each of the five areas provide a bar for the subject's individual score on the area, the average score in that area for all subjects from that organization, a bar for the subject's overall score, and a bar showing the 'benchmark.' The benchmark score is the average score in that area for all persons who have completed the instrument regardless of their organization. Finally, the report provides the strengths and areas for improvement according to the subject and according to all of the respondents.

Quantitative Findings of 360 Data

The quantitative data was subjected to a comparison of means between the PY1 baseline and the PY2 one year intervention data. The first analysis is a simple look at the overall mean scores on all five scales for the entire group. By the second program year only 29 of the supervisors who started in the first year remained in the project due to advancements and retirements. Table 1 shows the comparisons of the PY1 and PY2 results. Responses from all rating sources for all supervisors were subjected to a paired T-test analysis and differences were found to be statistically significant. The T-test value was 2.782 with 358 degrees of freedom, resulting in a significance of .006 (two tailed test with significance level of alpha = .05). Within the overall group, 19 supervisors' scores had improved while 10 had declined. This clearly show a mixed pattern of growth for some supervisors while others had declined in terms of the scores provided by all respondents–supervisors, peers and direct reports. The "Gap Analysis" displays graphically (see Figure 1) the pattern. Here it is interesting to note the close matching of the scores by areas of evaluation with the PY1 line being remarkably similar to the PY2 line.

When overall scores are compared to the external baseline data, the profile is exactly the same with manager and facilitator functions rating the lowest and communicator and professional the highest. The

TABLE 1. Mean Scale Scores by Rating Category
All Respondents PY1 vs PY2

	2003	2004	Difference
Communicator	419	428	9
Leader	411	424	13
Manager	397	407	10
Facilitator	409	421	12
Professional	425	437	12
Mean All Scales	412	423	11

Note: Means Scale Score are multiplied by 100 for clarity.

FIGURE 1. Gap Analysis All Respondents

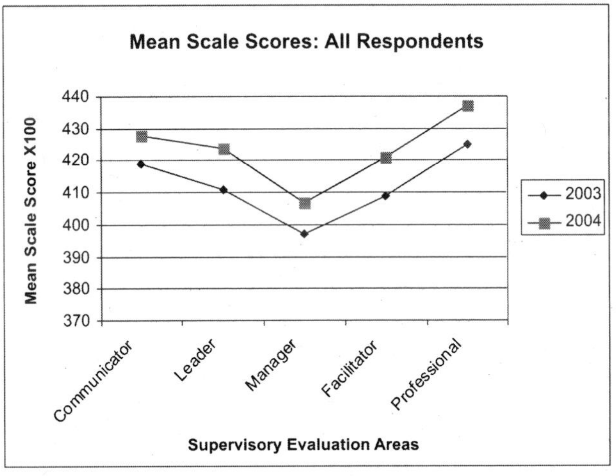

Missouri supervisors' scores on all items are significantly higher than those reported for the national baseline of comparable positions in like agencies.

As noted in the opening, the intervention model being tested here is concerned with how first line supervisors pass clinical skill and knowledge building along to their subordinates. Therefore the data provided by 'direct reports' would be of particular interest. Table 2 provides the group means scores by direct reports. Again all the differences show improvement on each scale from PY1 to PY2. All direct report responses for all supervisors were subjected to a paired T-test analysis and differences were found to be statistically significant. The T-test values was 3.5666 with 138 degrees of freedom resulting in significance greater than 1 in 1000 (significance >.000, two tailed test with alpha + .05). The gap analysis (see Figure 2) shows a very different pattern for PY2 than for PY1. The PY1 line for direct reports is remarkably similar to the pattern shown for all respondents in PY1. The PY2 scores show a different pattern with pronounced growth in the manager and facilitator roles and some growth in the professional roles. Clearly the direct reports are scoring their supervisors higher in these areas. The overall pattern shows 22 supervisors to have gained in the views of their workers. The gain from direct reports is offset in the overall score (cf. Table 1 and Figure 1) by a slight decrease in peer scores in the second rating period.

The data from PY1 and PY2 for all respondents and for direct reports only cannot be said to meet a rigorous standard of statistical significance. However, the overall improvement in scores from all respondents and the differing pattern from direct reports suggests that the supervisors were showing different patterns of behavior toward those they work with. The next section turns to more qualitative analysis.

TABLE 2. Mean Scale Scores by Rating Category Direct Report Respondents Only: PY1 vs PY2

	2003	2004	Difference
Communicator	420	436	16
Leader	413	433	20
Manager	402	434	32
Facilitator	410	448	38
Professional	418	442	24

Note: Means Scale Scores are multiplied by 100 for clarity.

FIGURE 2. Gap Analysis Direct Report Respondents

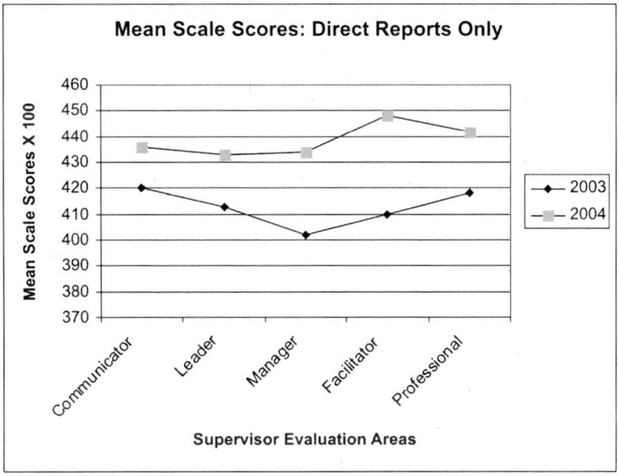

Individual Development Plan Results

The entire process of input, evaluation, feedback and interpretation of results that forms the core of the 360 process would be pointless unless it were coupled with an action phase building upon those data. As noted previously, the Individual Development Plan (IDP) is a critical aspect of employing this tool to produce behavioral and organizational change and the results further reinforce the comparative score data described above.

At the conclusion of the year 2003 feedback sessions, each supervisor developed an IDP that specified from one to four behavioral goals to be accomplished during the coming year along with action steps and resources required for achieving the objectives. The thirty-two participants and their managers together identified and agreed on 108 goals (m = 3.38) and the attendant steps, resources and timelines. A supervisor/ manager countersigned copy of each IDP was filed with research team. The goals determined by the participants were closely geared to the content of the adopted instrument but latitude was also provided for them to specify arenas of professional concern not addressed by this 30 items SOE form.

By the time of the second administration of the instrument the number of participants had decreased to twenty-nine though promotions and resignation. During the 2004 debriefing sessions, the IDP document was individually reviewed with each supervisor and their subjective assessment recorded. Subsequently an item comparison analysis linking the goals with instrument items was conducted. The mean score of the keyed items for the 2003 iteration of the 360 was 3.97 and that number increased to 4.17 in 2004. Twenty-one of the 29 remaining supervisors had an increased mean score on their particular constellation of behavioral aims. Scores ranged up to .78 higher while the range of lower scores was considerably lower. Interviews with participants who did not fare as well in the second administration pointed to a consistent pattern of staff unrest and labor-management problems in those offices and again illustrate the environmental sensitivity of 360 instruments discussed in a preceding section of this paper. Seventy-two percent of the unique behaviors targeted among all the supervisors showed improvement from the year one to the year two ratings. Table 3 lists the most commonly specified goals and the 360 scoring on those items in the first and second rating periods:

The first item is of particular interest in the overall evaluation of this project since the model of supervision being tested is "role demonstration" which requires the superiors to show techniques to their subordinates. Associated with this element is the structured feedback which, in these sites, was principally through regularly scheduled case conferences, a departure from the former practice of case consultation on an ad hoc basis. Organizational morale shows the greatest gain among the top six goals and this might be expected for an item that is actually an aggregate of many behavioral changes in an organization. The one goal in which respondent raters did not see growth among these supervisors was in the area of appropriate control of emotional response. Although

TABLE 3. Individual Development Plan Goals

Most Common IDP Goals			
Item	2003 score	2004 score	change +/–
Model practice for workers (14)	3.91	4.20	+.29
Provide structured feedback (12)	4.00	4.27	+.27
Sense of community/morale (12)	3.87	4.19	+.32
Better control of emotions (10)	4.21	4.00	–.21
Improved unit communication (10)	4.05	4.28	+.23
Work organization/time management (10)	3.93	4.07	+.14

the composite rating does not meet the standard for an "area of concern," the slippage is notable as a departure from an otherwise positive trend. Better work organization and time management may be linked to the perceived improvement in unit communications. Since the inception of this process most of the supervisors report that they have instituted regular group meetings within their units both for administrative purposes and as a medium for teaching clinical practice skills.

There are several caveats that must be mentioned in this study. The use of paired T-tests as the statistical procedure is limited here by the anonymity procedures in place. As workers come and go during a years time and as supervisors are moved to different units, pairing the observations is made more difficult. Workplace changes including interpersonal and work place tensions may also affect the ratings given to a specific individual. Overall the data is remarkably consistent is showing a pattern of improvement in supervisory performance judged by their superiors, peers and workers. Perhaps most important is that workers judged their supervisors to have improved in their performance in some critical areas.

IMPLICATIONS FOR PRACTICE

What lessons can then be learned from this study's results? First, when supervisors experience, many for the first time, a balanced assessment of their overall performance which is directed to their professional growth and the assessment is given in a growth enhancing manner, they often are empowered to improve their assessment and emphasis on growth of their workers. Second, evidence based practice requires a systematic method for judging how supervisors conduct themselves. The 360-degree evaluation, when carefully employed as a development tool, provides good 'evidence' for the evaluation of supervisory performance. When supervisors are evaluated by those who report to them a new dynamic of collegiality and mutual professionalism is established. Third, the 360 evaluation when coupled with feedback focused on the supervisor's own development provides a source of empowerment, refreshment, and support. These actions alone may reduce stress and burnout enabling the supervisory to have 'more to give' to their workers.

This experience does support the contention that specifically targeted supervisory behaviors can and do change when a developmental plan of action is designed and carried through and that having feedback data upon which to build clearly assists in focusing such action plans. However, it is also evident from this experience that managerial commitment and support for the supervisor is essential if the individual development plans are to achieve their intended aims. Where the IDP was viewed by management as an organizational contract to which the agency as well as the supervisor was committed, the results were significantly better.

Finally, once again organizational constraints are a significant confounding variable in attempting to modify the individual supervisor's practice. Project participants regularly report in debriefing interviews their frustration with the inability to make greater application of the training content and 360 feedback because of covering vacant caseloads, spending inordinate amounts of time and energy in new staff orientation and dealing with ad hoc accountability demands. While the 360 feedback process and its attendant developmental planning process can have a substantial impact on changing organizational culture in a child welfare agency, commitment of appropriate support from the controllers of all of the organization's resources is critical if it is to realize its potential for service improvement.

REFERENCES

Atwater, L., & Waldman, D. (1998). Accountability in 360 degree feedback. *Human Resource Magazine, 43*(6), 96-104.

Auteri, E. (1994). Upward feedback leads to culture change. *Human Resource Magazine*, (June), 78-84.

Barling, J., Wade, B., & Fullagar, C. (1990). Predicting employee commitment to company and union: divergent models. *Journal of Personnel Psychology, 63*(1), 49-63.

Bayfield, A.H., & Crocket, W.H. (1955). Employee attitudes and employee performance. *Psychological Bulletin, 52*, 396-424.

Blau, G. (1999). Testing the longitudinal impact of work variables and performance appraisal satisfaction on subsequent overall job satisfaction. *Human Relations, 52*(8), 1099-1113.

Bolm, C., Pettit, L. Kelly, M., & Wolchko, D. (2003). Evaluating Missouri CPS supervisory development project. *Professional Development, 6*(1), 68-73.

Brohl, K. (2004). *The New Miracle Workers: Overcoming Contemporary Challenges in Child Welfare Work.* Washington, DC: Child Welfare League of America.

Brooke, P., & Price, J. (1989). The determinants of absenteeism: An empirical test of a causal model. *Journal of Occupational Psychology, 62*(1), 1-19.

Casey Family Services. (2003). *Strengthening Families and Communities: Creative Strategies.* Baltimore, MD: Casey Family Services, Center for Effective Child Welfare Practice.

Child Welfare League of America. (2003). *Preventing Burnout in Your Staff and Yourself: A Survival Guide for Human Services Supervisors.* Washington, DC: Child Welfare League of America.

Child Welfare League of America. (2003) *The CWLA 2003 Salary Study*. Washington, DC: Child Welfare League of America.

Coggburn, J. (1998). Subordinate appraisals of managers: Lessons from a state agency. *Review of Public Personnel Administration, 18*(1), 68-79.

Daley, D. (1986). Humanistic management and organizational success: The effect of job and work environment characteristics on organizational effectiveness, public responsiveness, and job satisfaction. *Public Personnel Management, 15*, 131-142.

Ellett, A.J. (2001). Child welfare self-efficacy beliefs in two states: Implications for employee retention and practice. Paper presented at the Society for Social Work and Research 5th Annual Conference, Atlanta, Georgia.

Emmett, M., & Taher, W. (1992). Public sector professionals: The effects of public sector jobs on motivation, job satisfaction and work involvement. *American Review of Public Administration, 22*, 37-48.

Evans, G., Bryant, E. Owens, J., & Kelly, K. (2004). Ethnic differences in burnout, coping and intervention among childcare professionals. *Child and Youth Care Forum, 33*(5), 349-371.

Fleenor, J., & Prince, J. (1997). *Using 360-degree Feedback in Organizations: An Annotated Bibliography*. Greensboro, NC: Center for Creative Leadership. Ghorpade, J. (2000). Managing five paradoxes of 360-degree feedback. *The Academy of Management Executive, 14*(1), 140.

Hackman, J., & Lawler, E. (1971). Employee reaction to job characteristics. *Journal of Applied Psychology, 55*, 259-286.

Hackman, J., & Oldham, G. (1976). Motivation through the design of work: Test of a theory. *Organizational Behavior and Human Performance, 16*, 250-279.

Haworth, S. (1998). The dark side of multi-rater assessments. *Human Resource Magazine, 43*(6), 106-114.

Heathfield, S. (2001). 360 degree feedback: The good, the bad and the ugly. *Human Resources Newsletter*, (4/125/01) @ humanresources.about.com/cs/360 feedback.

Herzberg, F. (1968). One more time: How do you motivate employees? *Harvard Business Review, 46*, 53-62.

Hoffman, R. (1995). Ten reasons you should be using 360-degree feedback. *Human Resource Magazine, 40*(4), 82-85.

Iaffaldano, M., & Muchinsky, P. (1985). Job satisfaction and job performance: A meta-analysis. *Psychology Bulletin, 97*(2), 251-273.

Kadushin, A. (1992). *Supervision in Social Work (3rd. ed.)*. New York: Columbia University Press.

Kelly, M. (2001). Management mentoring in a social service agency. *Administration in Social Work, 25*(1), 17-33.

Kelly, M., & Lauderdale, M. (1999). Mentoring and organizational learning. *Professional Development: The International Journal of Continuing Social Work Education, 2*(3), 19-28.

Kirksey, J. (1994). Companies evaluate employees from all perspectives. *Personnel Journal, 11*, 92-94.

Kluger, A., & DeNisi, A. (1996). The effects of feedback interventions on performance: A historical review, a meta-analysis, and a preliminary feedback intervention. *Psychological Bulletin, 119*, 254-284.

Lauderdale, M. (1999) Reinventing Texas government. Austin, TX: University of Texas Press.

Lepsinger, R., & Lucia, A. (1997), 369 degree feedback and performance appraisal. *Training, 34*(9), 62-70.

Leslie, J., & Fleenor, J. (1998). *Feedback to Managers: A Review and Comparison of Multi-rater Instruments for Management Development.* Greensboro, NC: Center for Creative Leadership.

Lewis, G. (1987). Men and women toward the top: Backgrounds, careers and potential of federal middle managers. *Public Personnel Management, 21*, 473-491.

Likert, R. (1961). *New Patterns of Management.* New York: McGraw Hill.

Likert, R. (1967). *The Human Organization: In Management and Value.* New York: McGraw Hill.

Lind, C. (2004). Developing and supporting a continuum of child welfare services. *Welfare Information Network, 8*(6).

Lloyd, C., King, R. and Chenoweth, L. (2002). Social work, stress and burnout: A review. *Journal of Mental Health, 11*(3), 255-265.

London, M., Smither, J., & Adsit, D. (1997). Accountability: The Achilles' heel of multisource feedback. *Group and Organization Management, 22*(2), 162-184.

London, M., & Smithers, J. (1995). Can multi-source feedback change perceptions of goal accomplishment, self-evaluation, and performance-related outcomes? Theory-based application and directions for research. *Personnel Psychology, 48* (Winter), 803-839.

Maslow, A. (1954). *Motivation and Personality.* New York: Harper and Row.

McGregor, D. (1960). *The Human Side of Enterprise.* New York: McGraw Hill.

Mermelstein, J., & Sundet, P. (1978). A teaching model for rural field instruction. *Social Work in Rural Areas: Preparation and Practice.* Knoxville, TN: University of Tennessee.

Organ, D. (1988). A restatement of the satisfaction-performance hypothesis. *Journal of Management, 14*(4), 547-557.

Organizational Excellence Group: Leadership Tools (2000) accessed at www.utexas.edu/research/cswr/survey/site/leader/index.html

Orr, S. (1999). Child protection at the crossroads: Child abuse, child protection and recommendations for reform. *Policy Study No. 262.* Los Angeles: Reason Foundation.

Shama, J., McKelvey, J. Hardy, R., Epstein, M.H., Lomax, R.G., & Hurby, P.J. (1997). Job satisfaction of child welfare workers in an urban setting: Status and predictors. *Journal of Child and Family Studies, 6*(2), 209-219.

Pfau, B. (2002) Does 360-degree feedback negatively affect company performance? *Human Resource Magazine, 46*(6), 99-110.

Snell, L. (2000). Child welfare reform and the role of privatization. *Policy Study No. 271.* Los Angeles: Reason Foundation.

Stevens, M., & Higgins, D.J. (2002). The influence of risk and protection factors on burnout experienced by those who work with maltreated children. *Child Abuse Review, 11*(5), 313-331.

Sugrue, B. (2003). *State of the Industry.* Alexandria, VA: American Society of Training and Development.

Sundet, P., & Cowger, C. (1990). Rural community environment as a stress factor for rural child welfare workers. *Administration in Social Work, 14*(3).

Sundet, P., & Cowger, C. (2003) *Missouri Public Sector: A Market Comparison Study*. Columbia, MO: University of Missouri-Columbia.

Sundet, P., Mermelstein, J., & Watt, J.W. (2003). The role demonstration model of supervision. *Professional Development, 6*(1), 60-67.

Taylor, D. (1999). Managing job satisfaction. *Australian CPA, 69*(9), 46-49.

Ting, Y. (1996). Analysis of job satisfaction of the federal white-collar work force: Finding from the survey of federal employees. *American Review of Public Administration, 26*(4), 439-456.

U.S. Merit Systems Protection Board. (1990). *Working for America: A Federal Employee Survey*. Washington, DC: Government Printing Office.

U.S. Office of Personnel Management. (1997). *360-degree Assessment: An Overview*. McLean, VA: Human Technology, Inc.

Wagner, R., van Reyk, P., & Spence, N. (2001). Improving the working environment for workers in children's welfare agencies. *Child and Family Social Work, 6*(2), 161-178.

Waldman, D., & Atwater, L. (1998). *The Power of 360 Feedback: How to Leverage Performance Evaluations for Top Productivity*. Huston: Gulf Publishing.

Warrick, S. (1992). Supervisor review sheds light on blind spots. *Human Resource Magazine*, June, 111-120.

Wimer, S., & Nowack, S. (1998). 13 common mistakes using 360-degree feedback. *Training and Development, 52*(5), 288-309.

doi:10.1300/J394v04n03_10

Agency-Academic Collaboration in Evidence-Based Practice: A Case Example in Data Driven Innovation

Paul Sundet, PhD
Michael J. Kelly, PhD

SUMMARY. Evidence-based practice requires special expertise and ideological commitment which are harder to operationalize than to articulate. Combining the elements of a learning community with the research orientation required of an evidence-based approach to innovation led the authors to revisit the Intervention Design and Development model posited by Rothman and others. Applying it to a staff development initiative provides evidence that an interstitial system composed of academics and agency personnel, drawing on the unique talents and contributions of each, can work together in improving the quality of practice while simultaneously meeting the separate needs of each constituency. doi:10.1300/J394v04n03_11 *[Article copies available for a fee from The Haworth Document Delivery Service: 1-800-HAWORTH. E-mail address: <docdelivery@haworthpress.com> Website: <http://www.HaworthPress.com> © 2007 by The Haworth Press, Inc. All rights reserved.]*

Paul Sundet is affiliated with School of Social Work, University of Missouri-Columbia

Michael J. Kelly is affiliated with School of Social Work, University of Missouri-Columbia

[Haworth co-indexing entry note]: "Agency-Academic Collaboration in Evidence-Based Practice: A Case Example in Data Driven Innovation." Sundet, Paul and Michael J. Kelly. Co-published simultaneously in the *Journal of Evidence-Based Social Work* (The Haworth Press, Inc.) Vol. 4, No. 3/4, 2007, pp. 163-182; and: *Developing an Empirically Based Practice Inititative: A Case Study in CPS Supervision* (ed: Jenny L. Jones, and Paul Sundet) The Haworth Press, 2007, pp. 163-182. Single or multiple copies of this article are available for a fee from The Haworth Document Delivery Service [1-800-HAWORTH, 9:00 a.m. - 5:00 p.m. (EST). E-mail address: docdelivery@haworthpress.com].

Available online at http://jebsw.haworthpress.com

doi:10.1300/J394v04n03_11

KEYWORDS. Collaboration, practice development, academic/agency coordination, program evaluation, public child welfare

INTRODUCTION

The case for empirically validated practice in social work has been made for a number of years and by some of the most illustrious scholars that the profession has produced (Dawes, 1994; Thyer & Wodarski, 1998; Wodarski & Thyer, 1998: Roberts & Yeager, 2004). However, an equally learned and vociferous community of practitioners decries the reliance on a positivist stance and argues for the uniqueness of the individual experience and an interpretism rather than a positivism stance as core to the profession (cf. descriptions in Allen-Meares & DeRoos, 1994; Gibbs & Gambrill, 2002). The issue has likewise been joined in the field of child welfare and the advocates are often doctrinaire and strident (Barratt, 2003; Chaffin & Friedlich, 2004; Dawson & Berry, 2002; English, Bradford & Coghlan, 2000; Usher & Wildfire, 2003). But increasingly there are those who seek to bring the polar positions into harmony under the umbrella concept of evidence-based practice. Elsewhere in this journal the case for an evidence-based model has been made in detail by several authors (Collins-Camargo, 2005; Shackelford, et al. 2005) as well works previously cited. To those substantial contributions the authors would emphasize two critical rationales for this approach. The first is founded on professionalism and the second pragmatism, both values long held in this field.

The ethical foundation for evidence based practice is found in the code of ethics of all the helping professions. In social work and social services it is based on two core values, integrity and competence. The relevant statements from the National Association of Social Workers (NASW) Code of Ethics (1999) are: "Social workers should base practice on recognized knowledge, including empirically based knowledge relevant to social work and social work ethics" (Code 4.01) and "Social workers should critically examine and keep current with emerging knowledge relevant to social work and use evaluation and research evidence in their professional practice" (Code 5.02) The very nature of who the profession is and professes to be demands that practice be from a scientifically validated and reliable data foundation. Compelling support for this position can be found in both Gambrill (2004) who examines how practitioners can meet these obligations and Thyer (2004) who argues for even stronger guidelines of this nature in social work ethics.

The second reason may be somewhat cynically characterized as "survival." The field is faced with increased demand for services with shrinking resources, an ever greater number and variety of safety and well-being issues, varying definitions of appropriate agency role and action, conflicts in public policy approaches, rapid turnover in the workforce and a generalized belief that intervention does not work. Systematic accumulation of defensible evidence is required to answer all of these survival issues (Rosen, 2003).

However, even if one accepts that evidence-based practice is critical to child welfare, there still remains the core question of "how" such an approach can be practically implemented. In this article we take the position that developing a learning community is essential and that this can most effectively be accomplished by combining the unique assets of the service delivery agency and the academic institution in an interstitial structure that capitalizes on the strengths of each to their mutual benefit. Data from such an experiment will be provided to illustrate this proposition.

EVIDENCE-BASED PRACTICE

There are multiple definitions of evidence-based practice as well as a variety of terms that are somewhat loosely used interchangeably with it. For our purposes the operational definition we use is as follows: Evidence-based practice is a type of intervention in which the professional uses research as a practice and problem solving tool; collects data systematically to monitor intervention; specifies problems, techniques and outcomes in measurable terms; and systematically evaluates the effectiveness of the interventions used. The goal is to use the best evidence to guide interventions that will benefit the client, enhance the quality and outcomes of care, and be cost effective (Illinois MISA Institute, 2001).

Although most of the literature written on this subject focuses the concept on analysis of techniques and outcomes of direct one-on-one intervention in the counseling and/or behavioral change arena, we would argue that empirically-based practice has at least equal relevance at other systemic levels of intervention (Simpson, 2002). The authors' working definition of "practice" encompasses the domains of policy formulation, program design, administration, procedure development and organizational resource control as well as direct client clinical intervention. And empirically-based practice can and must take place at micro (individual case load) mezzo (unit/office) and macro (agency-wide) levels. In fact, the same phenomenon often needs to be addressed at the all three levels simultaneously if practice is to be effective

Learning Organization

In a child welfare system that aspires to be data-driven and evidence-based there are a number of conditions that must be meet and adhered to Included in that list is openness to reviewing current policy and practice, readiness to give up "top-down" decision making, willingness to connect with the local reality and to make appropriate data available to the community decision makers. Learning organizations are environments where people continually expand their capacity to create results they truly desire, where new and expansive patterns of thinking are nurtured, collective aspirations are set free and where people are continually learning together. Among the essential conditions of a learning community are continuous development opportunities, the use of learning to reach defined goals, the linking of organization and individual performance and fostering inquiry and dialogue and making it safe for people to share openly and take risks. Consequences of these conditions include creative tension as a source of energy and renewal and a conscious awareness of and interaction with the practice context. Several of these imperatives have been explored by Kelly and Lauderdale (1999, 2001).

Integrative Model

Obviously incorporating both essential elements of evidence-based practice and a learning community in to a model of intervention, while clearly compatible and desirable, is no easy task (Lehman, Greener & Simpson, 2002). The aim is nothing less than achieving an environment in which research methodology can be explicitly focused on creating, expanding and enhancing the tools of professional practice. Substantial literature exists that has historically offered approaches to this issue (Rothman, 1980, Reid, 1987, Fairfield, 1967, Baker & Schultz, 1971; Thomas 1978). But much of the methodological literature on the subject is dichotomous. There is research *about* practice which has been traditionally the province of the academy and research *for* practice which has most often arisen from the service delivery systems. Both are essential and need not be mutually exclusive. And, in fact, it is our contention that neither is complete without the other. One approach to integrating these two somewhat differing streams is known as Intervention Design and Development (Rothman, 1989).

Rothman defines Intervention Design and Development (ID&D) as "sequential and interconnected activities that culminate in the creation of innovative intervention tools" (Rothman, 1992, p. 52).

The central mission of ID&D is the production of reliable, knowledge-driven methods of intervention. The focus is on the pragmatic, the utilitarian, the practical solving of pressing practice issues. Both effectiveness of action and efficiency of resource use are of concern. Knowledge development is a by-product of the problem-solving rather than an end goal in itself. This model assumes an on-going, coordinated and sequentially repetitive series of activities to create a coherent whole that is empirically based practice.

The stages begin with data driven needs assessment using techniques beyond but not abandoning the usual methods of key informant and expert opinion. Social indicator data, rate-under-treatment, community forum and social survey procedures take central roles to buttress (or contradict) the prevailing professional opinion.

Library science and Meta-analysis are key ingredients in both expanding and circumscribing the purview of inquiry and the range of alternatives to be considered. Expertise in the technology of data search is an indispensable tool at this level. Techniques may range from the mundane review of the literature to the esoteric statistical analysis.

Design, management and constant up-dating of a management information system is a core element to the ID&D process which requires systematic data bases as the raw material from which to construct the field experiments which follow.

Field experiments, using a wide range of methodologies, pilot proposed solutions in controlled environments in which as many intervening variables as possible in a real-life situation are accounted for. Creative construction of the experiments, use of multiple forms of design and foresight in isolating contaminating factors are essential ingredients at this stage.

Pilots are dispassionately evaluated for what they tell about both process and outcome in the experimental sites. What has not succeeded is as carefully analyzed as the purported "successes" for it is from the former that the most valuable lessons are often gleaned.

Diffusion studies and marketing research that draw on the business world comprise the final components of this overall research enterprise. The latter are often neglected in the public sector but have both as much utility and as much importance as they do in the profit-making arenas. A solidly grounded intervention in a field like child welfare may simply not be politically feasible in a given environment or a given time, irrespective of the empirical evidence that supports its effectiveness. The resulting strategy of intervention may be one of political/public education as a precursor to introducing a clinical strategy.

ID&D incorporates a number of already existing methods and integrates them into a sequential and coherent program that applies a research mentality as well as technique to answering in a real-time context the critical practice and policy questions faced by the child welfare agency.

First and foremost there must be an organizational commitment to empirically based decision making beginning with identification of issues and problems. A second requirement is the development of an internal infrastructure to support a research orientation. A true internal "research shop" needs to exist having the capability of oversight, direction and design authority for various initiatives that administration may wish to undertake. This requires a specific allocation of funds and positions to perform both the enhanced MIS and the research functions.

A third element is developing an organizational culture in which all levels within the structure have an appreciation for and an expectation that research-generated data will the touchstone from which practice decisions are made. This includes the acculturation of employees through the immediate supervisory structure that reinforces the evidence based mind set and special attention must be paid to making research findings practical and beneficial to the front-line staff.

The fourth required component is a careful analysis of what functions are best performed within the agency and those that may require the unique expertise of an external resource. The depth of specialized expertise required in some components of ID&D model can most efficiently be accessed through a collaborative arrangement with a community of scholars who share the same superordinate goals and value orientation. Each side to such an arrangement brings unique talents, knowledge and perspectives which can inform and refine the research enterprise. And each can benefit, both in terms of the overarching objective and in achieving their unique mission-driven goals.

INTERSTITIAL SYSTEM ELEMENTS

Developing an interstitial system that encompasses the disparate elements of the child welfare delivery system and the varieties of interests in the academy can be a daunting task. Briar-Lawson and Zlotnick (2003) in their recent work point to many of the opportunities and difficulties that exist and make a significant contribution by going beyond academic degree program collaboration to explore broader arenas of professional commonality.

The Intervention Design and Development (ID&D) model detailed above illustrates how the strengths-based ideology the child welfare field prides itself on can meld together two somewhat entities to build upon the unique assets of each and, simultaneously, meet their separate and distinct goals.

The first step, needs assessment, is the province of both the agency's direct client interface and the academy's experts in applied research technologies. Often initial needs assessment is primarily anecdotal and while qualitative perceptions gathered from practitioners in the field have substantial merit in assessing needs, other and more scientifically rigorous methods are also required to justify resource expenditure and disruption of current organization practice.

Meta analysis is a particular asset of those with formal academic training in research methods. Not only have faculty been educated to the nuisances of such analysis, they frequently have access to information resources and an available infrastructure for detailed program and evaluation searches that most agencies do not.

Conversely, the management information service is the particular strength the agency brings to the ID&D enterprise. All design and development assumes the existence of a critical information baseline from which comparison methodologies and impact studies flow. Without such an MIS in place, the process of design is both arduous and haphazard. Academic expertise can be of value in a consultative role to the agency in this area but primary responsibility for a current and appropriate data reporting structure rests with the child welfare agency and is a sine qua non for this collaboration to move forward effectively.

In field experiments, each partner brings uniqueness. The agency has access to the client-worker interface where essential data will be generated and provides the legal auspices and sanction for intervention. Often, too, the agency has the necessary credibility with the clientele and parallel agencies to initiate innovation although it is not uncommon the prestige of the academic institution is a major advantage in instituting change, particularly when it constitutes significant departure from past practices. The academy brings detailed knowledge of research design, potential contaminates and data analysis techniques not commonly available internally in child welfare agencies.

A critical element the interstitial system provides is a dispassionate approach to analysis. Pilots are often and naturally the "fair-haired child" of program administrators who have invested intellectual and emotional capital as well as monetary resources in an idea. Facing a less than favorable outcome takes fortitude that is bolstered by what Lawson et al. (2003) have termed the "design team," a combination of agency and academic personnel working in collaboration over time.

The final element of the model is diffusion and marketing. External diffusion through professional publication is the life blood of the academic and meets survival requirements for the individual faculty member and institutional maintenance needs for sponsoring departments and colleges. The promise of such diffusion opportunities is a major motivating factor for academics to invest in the ID&D process. Internal diffusion relies on the effectiveness and openness of the agency's internal communication structure. Marketing a new intervention design is frequently a political process and while the agency has a special responsibility in this area, the academy offers unique expertise found in a range of disciplines that can be mobilized to assist in design and execution of communications targeted to specific audiences.

"DOUBLE LOOP" LEARNING AND THE ID&D PROCESS

While the ID&D model provides the practical application for evidence based practice, the theoretical support depends upon organizational learning. Argyris and Schön's (1978, p. 2-8) learning theory asserts that most organizational learning is based in "error detection" and corrective actions that attempt to return the organizational to the status quo. These actions they call 'single loop' learning. An unfortunate aspect of single loop learning is that it fosters avoidance of ideas which challenge cherished beliefs and often provoke defensive reactions to criticism. Single loop learning never challenges the organization's underlying assumptions, organizational methods, or its objectives. For example, child welfare systems throughout the US are challenged by a number of problems related to staff turnover and turnover's effect on service quality. The most common reaction is to assume these problems are the result of work that is inherently too difficult and that there is a lack of public understanding or support.

By contrast, 'double loop' learning occurs when deviations from acceptable standards of quality, i.e., 'errors,' are detected and the correction methods include modifications of the system's "governing variables"–its most deeply held values, beliefs and assumptions. Double loop learning requires that an organization gather valid information and hold an internal commitment to consideration of choices which may challenge the status quo. Double loop learning requires a more transparent organizational system which includes sharing control with key participants outside the organization, surfacing differences in values and opinions within the organization, a more open participation in program design and implementation, and a commitment to public testing of evaluations.

Like the ID&D process, double loop learning, is predicated on mutual trust, acceptance of one another's' expertise, subject matter credibility and an appreciation for the unique needs of each. It is difficult but it is also essential to maximize the resources required for good child welfare practice.

A SYSTEM IN OPERATION

A recent local example of the collaboration between the agency and the academy is a project entitled the Role Demonstration Model of CPS Supervision. This a classic example of the ID&D design, the complimentary roles that the service delivery agency and the academy can play in attaining a mutually desirable goal and incorporates essential elements of both evidence-based practice and a learning community.

The concern for clinical practice competence and most specifically for that competence among first-line supervisors has been voiced for a number of years by Missouri system administrators. The budget shortfalls of the past several years and the need to deliver basic orientation and training to new employees because of high turnover have made this emphasis on the supervisors reluctantly take a back seat. However, with a 2003 Children's Bureau (CB) initiative through the Southeastern Regional Quality Improvement Center–University of Kentucky College of Social Work, the opportunity arose to submit a competitive proposal for 42 months of funding to design and evaluate a training protocol specific to child protective services supervisors. A joint team of Missouri Children's Division and University of Missouri-Columbia School of Social Work personnel carefully examined the RFP and debated whether it was worth the substantial joint effort needed to undertake this complex a project with limited funding and scope. Ultimately the decision was made to go forward and the proposal was successful. From the very outset that original team has remained substantially in place and constitutes the Policy Board that exercises the oversight function including examining progress, content, policies and project outcomes. Sub-groups take on curriculum and research design responsibilities under aegis of the Board.

Throughout the process the decision-making was a joint venture. For instance, it was decided early on that "creaming" wasn't going to tell the system anything about the effectiveness of the intervention in modifying organizational practice and client outcomes. And so instead of taking volunteers from throughout the state as participants, the Board chose to pick two entire organizational units and take all of the supervisors (the good, the bad, and the indifferent) as experimental subjects. That meant including 35 participants rather than the 20 the CB protocol called for. The grant also specified a comparison group which was correspondingly expanded.

The project required that the applicant posit a specific model of supervision. Instead of turning first to the standard literature and picking an author, the Board relied on the internal needs assessment data that the agency had been gathering through employee feedback. Immediately it became evident that the major deficit noted by workers and supervisors alike was not in their basic training but in the absence of modeling practice skills in the work environment. Over 80% of the line staff expressed this need and over 65% noted that it was the most notable lack in their training. Associated with this finding were case analysis data gleaned from the Peer Record Review process that reported while safety issues were regularly addressed (92% timely first contact; 93% timely reports), in less than 40% of the cases was there evidence that the family was a participant in the case planning process and in just over half (51%) of the cases there was no clear service delivery plan with specific rather than generalized goals. These data combined to lead to a role demonstration approach with an emphasis on solution-focused brief therapy as a clinical model consistent with the already existing agency emphasis on family centered and strengths-based perspectives (Sundet, Mermelstein & Watt, 2003).

The research design was turned over to a joint team headed by a senior faculty member with substantial child welfare background and the chief of research/MIS for the agency. Additional members from both structures were added to round out the necessary expertise. The first principle adopted was to be as non-intrusive as possible but to measure as many variables as practical. This was significantly aided by the sophistication of the agency data systems that were already in place (Bolm et al., 2003). The following are the components being measured in the project at this time.

OUTCOME EXAMPLES

Measuring Organizational Change

The ID&D system discussed here is based in the use of instrumentation which has established uses within the child welfare system. Knowing that improvements in clinical supervision would likely require changes in the culture and climate of the organization, the Survey of Organizational Excellence (SOE) was selected to measure these aspects. The SOE has been used by the Children's' Division since 2002 as part of its quality improvement process. The instrument, designed to measure changes in organizational culture in five organizational dimensions (work group; accommodations; organizational features; information; personal demands), consisting of 20 constructs that are critical to organizational coherence, effectiveness and efficiency. Reliability and validity of the SOE were established during development. The constructs have adequate reliability (Cronbach's Alpha averaging .85).

The policy board (design team) from the agency and the university designated four SOE constructs that could measure changes in climate/culture. Four constructs falling within the personal demands dimension included job satisfaction, time/stress management, burnout, and empowerment. The team also selected the "employee development" construct. Two graphs compare the urban intervention (one judicial circuit) with the urban comparison (one judicial circuit) and the eight (8) rural intervention circuits covering 23 counties and six (6) rural comparison circuits covering 18 counties.

Graph OC 1 shows the comparison between the rural intervention circuits (noted here as experimental or Exp) and the rural comparison circuits (noted here as 'control'). No statistical differences in means (T-tests with alphas = .05) were found between the intervention circuits and the contrast circuits. The rural circuit's scores improved in all five measures between FY03 and FY04 and are higher than the contrast circuits in all measures except employee development. Graph OC2 shows the comparison between the urban intervention and the urban comparison circuits. No statistical differences in means (T-tests with alphas = .05) were found between the intervention and control circuits. However, within the urban intervention circuit, job satisfaction scores were significantly higher (alpha =.05) and all the other measures except employee development approached statistical significance at the .05 level. Again the scores show the urban intervention circuit's improvement over the contrast circuit on each measure except employee development.

CHART 1. OC1: Org. Culture Rural Circuits Exp vs Controls Baseline Yr2 vs First Intervention Year

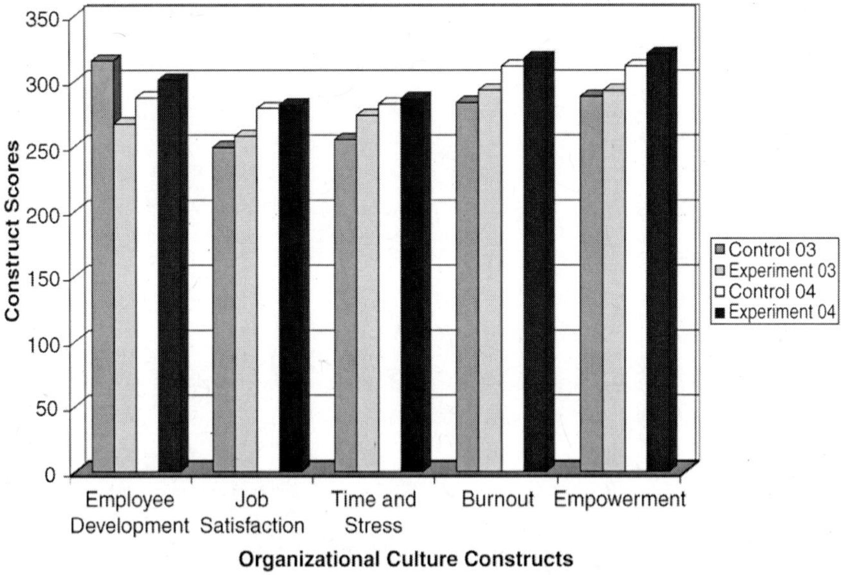

CHART 2. OC2: Urban Circuits Organizational Culture Baseline Yr2 vs First Intervention Year

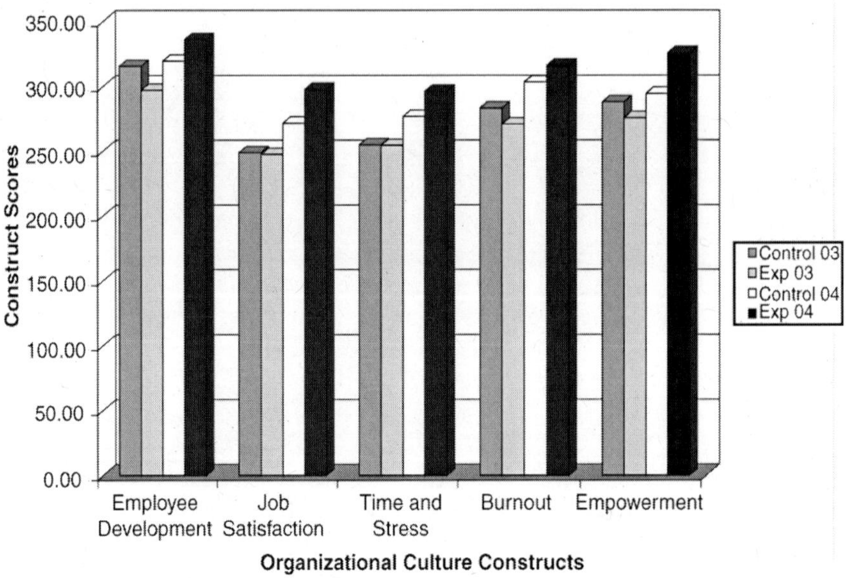

The design team also chose to measure the SOE construct "supervisory effectiveness." Graphs SE1 and SE2 which follow compare supervision in the intervention and contrast areas. The titles 'experiment' and 'control' are used to simplify reading of the graph material. In SE1, the rural circuit's data shows that the intervention circuits started the second baseline year (FY03) with a lower score than the control circuits but by the first intervention year (FY04) had significantly improved on this measure among themselves. This change is statistically significant at the Alpha = .05 level where a change of 50 points of the graph approximates statistical significance. The control circuits had also improved by FY04 but the experimental circuits were now scoring higher. While the intervention circuits did not score significantly higher statistically, the improvement is clear.

Graph SE2 shows the data for the Urban experimental and control circuits. In these graphs, a similar situation is seen. The urban intervention circuits scored lower than the control in FY03 but had improved dramatically by FY04. The control circuit changed far less between FY03 and FY04. While not statistically significant, the improvement in supervisory effectiveness is clear.

The design team concluded that because of the project expected to produce and measure organizational rather than individual change, measurement would be more difficult than in a more simplistic matched pairs model. However, these data are highly significant in that the experimental sites show positive change on every measure that was originally hypothesized to improve as a result of the intervention and the growth is dramatic when contrasted with the comparison sites; worker satisfaction with supervisory performance is substantially higher as is worker perception of supervisors' capability/effectiveness.

Measuring Changes in Child Welfare Outcomes

Again, in keeping with the ID&D model, the team chose also to depend upon measuring changes in the outcomes for children as measured by the Children's Division. Among the measures chosen, two are discussed here for illustrative purposes. First, measuring improvement in the timeliness of report completion and, below, reoccurrence of abuse in family centered cases.

State statute and agency policy dictates completion of child abuse and neglect investigation/assessment within 30 days of receipt of a report. This measure is calculated for child abuse and neglect reports concluded

CHART 3. (*a*) SE1: Supervisory Effectiveness Rural Circuits Second Baseline Year vs First Intervention Year; (*b*) SE2: Supervisory Effectiveness Urban Circuits Baseline Yr 2 vs First Intervention Yr

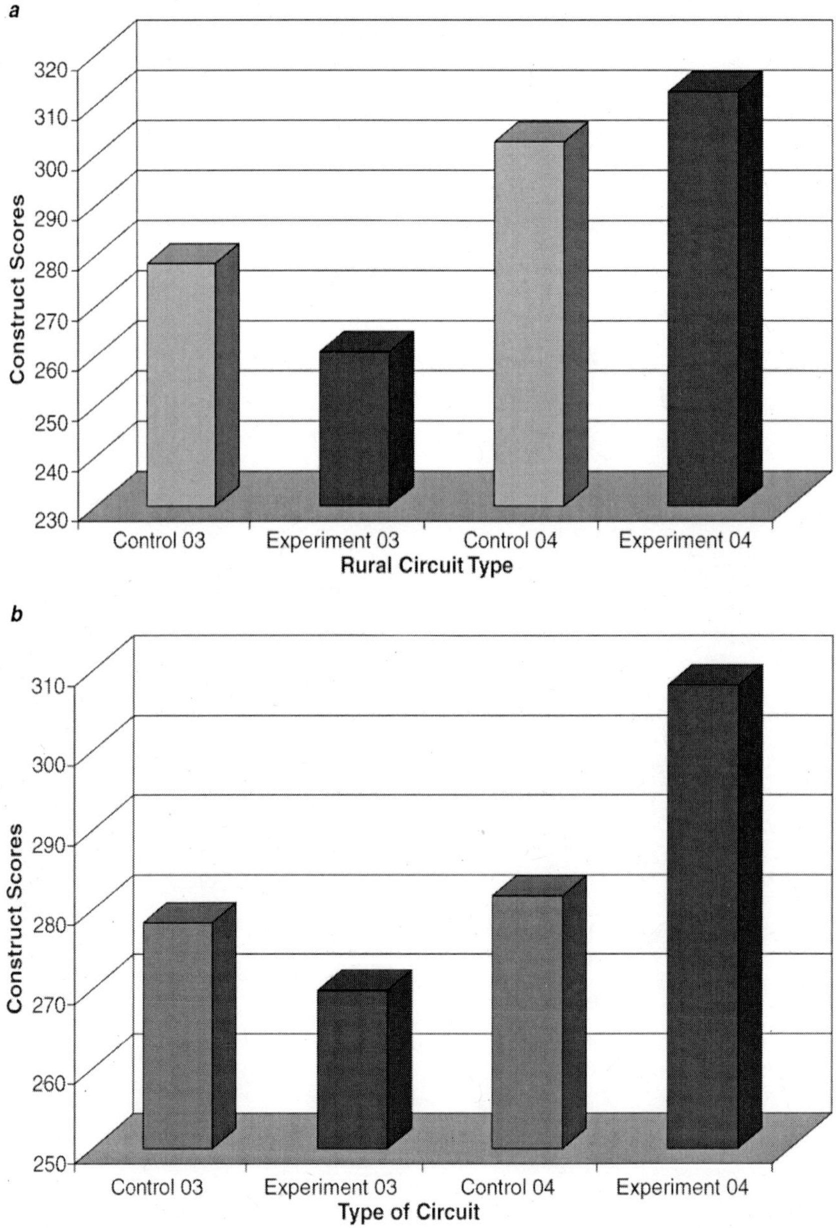

within the three month period under review. As seen in Figure 1, the proportion of case workers in the rural intervention region who completed a report within 30 days appears to have diminished, between Baseline Year I, with 60 percent meeting this performance standard in Intervention Year I. Within the urban region, case worker performance on this measure, as indicated by the trend line (marked on the charts as "linear"), suggests improvement (see Figure 2), with reports being completed within 30 days among more than 50 percent of the time.

These data suggest the importance of both the ID&D process and 'double loop' learning. The design team's discussion of the findings lead to consideration of one important aspect of the measurement which had not been initially considered. The RDM model being taught to the supervisors stresses improvements in case work. Improvements included more careful documentation and more intensive scrutiny of the individuals' cases and the family situations. The suggested improvements in case psycho-social background, more careful strength based diagnosis and more complete treatment planning all require more time on the part of the case workers. It is possible that as the RDM model is fully implemented 'timeliness of completion' will decline. This finding opens the door to a discussion of the 'governing variables' behind the measurement.

The second area chosen for illustration of the outcome measures concerns reduction of recurrence of abuse for family-centered care cases. This measure provides the percentage of children in Family-Centered

FIGURE 1. Timeliness of Completion of Reports

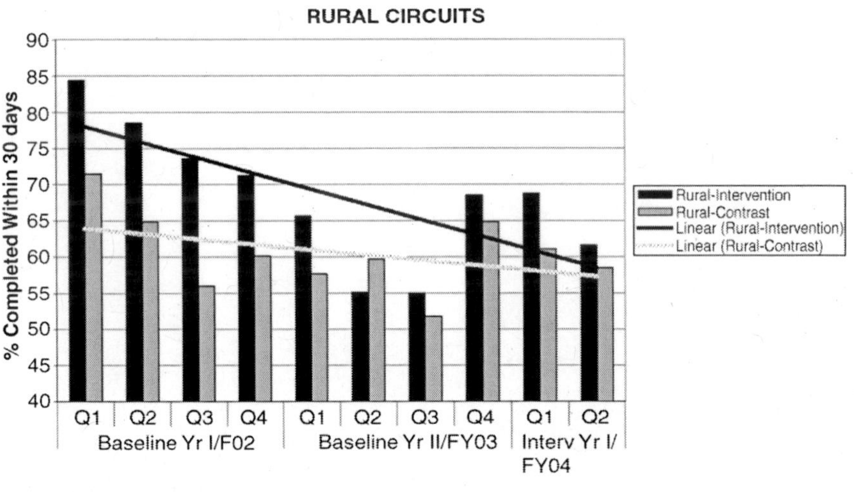

Services cases who remain in intact families with a substantiated child abuse and neglect report within the three month period under review. Within the rural intervention region, this proportion diminished between Baseline Year I and Intervention Year I: less than 1.5 percent of the intact families had a subsequent substantiated child abuse and neglect report by the last time measured (Figure 3). As shown in Figure 4, in the urban

FIGURE 2. Timeliness of Completion of Reports

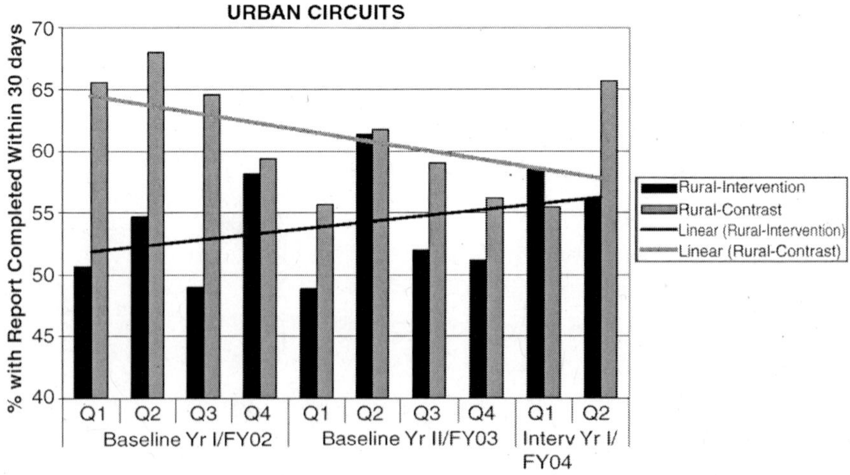

FIGURE 3. Recurrence of Abuse among Family-Centered Cases

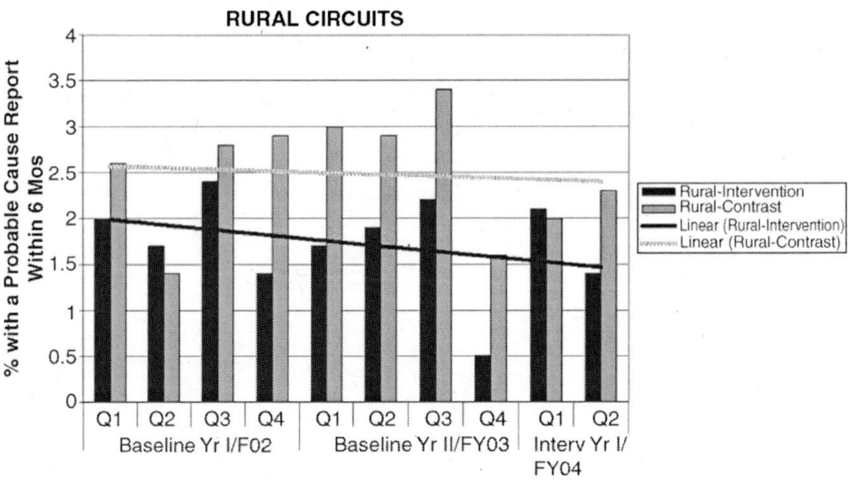

FIGURE 4. Recurrence of Abuse Among Family-Centered Cases

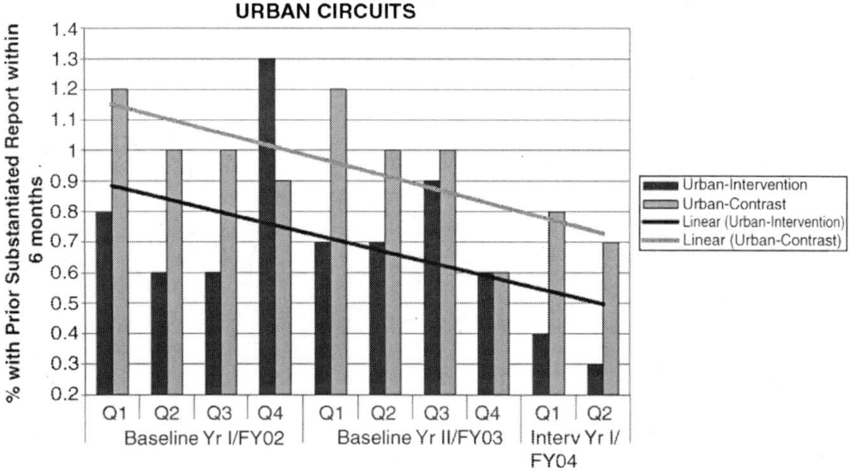

intervention area the proportion also diminished, with less than 0.3 percent of the intact families having a substantiated child abuse and neglect report made. Further analysis as the project proceeds is expected to demonstrate similar reductions.

Practice Modifications

Based on the results that this demonstration project has achieved in the first two years of its operation, several significant modifications have taken place within the state child welfare agency. First in the demonstration sites and now throughout the system, clinical performance expectations have been instituted for supervisors. Here-to-fore performance standards had been specified only in policy, procedure and administrative management functions. By adding this new category the agency officially recognizes that teaching clinical practice skills is a core aspect of the supervisor's job and, by implication, that the worker is expected to function as a behavioral change agent, not simply in surveillance and control capacities. A second impact associated with the first is rethinking and orienting the agency staff training and development paradigm. The focus had been on job specific techniques taught primarily from a technician stand point. The new approach emphasizes the professionalism of the staff at all levels and takes a personal developmental stance. The use of individual development plans that are contractually arrived at is spreading from the experimental sites to the other regions of the state. At the top management level there is a much stronger recognition of the utility of evidence-based intervention and commitment to systematic evaluation of programs. The agency is collaborating with the School on other design and demonstration initiatives based on this experience. Finally, among the project participants themselves there is a strong sense of professionalism and self-confidence based on not only the learning experiences they have had but also from the systematic feedback that they are receiving about the impact that their behaviors are having on worker performance and client outcomes.

PRACTICE MODIFICATIONS ACHIEVED

Based on the results that this demonstration project has achieved in the first two years of its operation, several significant modifications have taken place within the state child welfare agency. First in the demonstration sites and now throughout the system, clinical performance expectations have been instituted for supervisors. Here-to-fore performance standards had been specified only in policy, procedure and administrative management functions. By adding this new category the agency officially recognizes that teaching clinical practice skills is a core aspect of the supervisor's job and, by implication, that the worker is expected to function as a behavioral change agent, not simply in surveillance and control capacities. A second impact associated with the first is rethinking and orienting the agency staff training and development paradigm. The focus had been on job specific techniques taught primarily from a technician stand point. The new approach emphasizes the professionalism of the staff at all levels and takes a personal developmental stance. The use of individual development plans that are contractually arrived at is spreading from the experimental sites to the other regions of the state. At the top management level there is a much stronger recognition of the utility of evidence-based intervention and commitment to systematic evaluation of programs. The agency is collaborating with the School on other design and demonstration initiatives based on this experience. Finally, among the project participants themselves there is a strong sense of professionalism and self-confidence based on not only the learning experiences they have had but also from the systematic feedback that they are receiving about the impact that their behaviors are having on worker performance and client outcomes.

BIBLIOGRAPHY

Allen-Meares, P. & DeRoos, Y.Y. (1994). Are practitioner intuition and empirical evidence equally valid sources of professional knowledge? In W.W. Hudson & P.S. Nurius (Eds.). *Controversial Issues in Social Work Research*. Boston: Allyn & Bacon.

Argyris, C., & Schön, D. (1978) Organizational learning: A theory of action perspective. Reading, Mass: Addison Wesley.

Barker, R., & Schultz, R. (1971). *Instructional Product Development*. New York: Von Nostrand Reinhold Co.

Barratt, M. (2003). Organizational support for evidence-based practice within child and family social work: A collaborative study. *Child & Family Social Work, 8*(2), 143-151.

Bolm C., Pettit, L., & Kelly, M. (2003). Evaluating Missouri cps supervisory development project. *Professional Development, 6*(2), 68-73.

Briar-Lawson, K., & Zlotnick, J. (2003). *Charting the Impacts of University-Child Welfare Collaboration*. New York: Haworth Press.

Chaffin, M., & Friedlich, B. (2004). Evidence-based treatments in child abuse and neglect. *Children and Youth Services Review, 26*, 1097-1113.

Collins-Camargo, C. (2005). Administering research and demonstration projects aimed at promoting evidence-based practice in child welfare: Challenges and rewards. *Journal of Evidence Based Social Work* (this issue).

Dawes, R.M. (1994). *House of Cards: Psychology and Psychotherapy Built on Myth*. New York: Free Press.

Dawson, K., & Berry, M. (2002). Engaging families in child welfare services: An evidence–based approach to best practice. *Child Welfare, 81*(2), 293-317.

English, D.J., Bradford, C.C., & Coghlan, L. (2000). Data-based organizational change: The use of administrative data to improve child welfare programs and policy. *Child Welfare, 79*(5), 499-516.

Fairweather, G.W. (1967). *Methods for Experimental Innovation*. New York: John Wiley.

Gambrill, E. (2004). Contributions of critical thinking and evidence-based practice to the fulfillment of the ethical obligations of professionals. In H. Briggs & T. Rzepnicki (Eds.). *Using Evidence in Social Work Practice*. Chicago, IL: Lyceum Books.

Gibbs, L. & Gambrill, E. (2002). Evidence-based practice: Counterarguments to objections. *Research on Social Work Practice, 12*(3), 452-477.

Illinois MISA Institute (2001). Evidence-Based Practices in Mental Health (on-line article). University of Chicago Center for Psychiatric Rehabilitation. http://www.illionimisainstitute.org/library/article-evidence-based practices.

Kelly, M., & Lauderdale, M. (2001). Public private mentoring for leadership and service quality. *Professional Development: The International Journal of Continuing Social Work Education, 4*(2), 32-41.

Kelly, M., & Lauderdale, M. (1999). Mentoring and organizational learning. *Professional Development: The International Journal of Continuing Social Work Education, 2*(3), 19-28.

Lawson, H., Anderson-Butcher, D., Petersen, N., & Barkdull, C. (2003). Design teams as learning systems for complex systems change: Evaluation data and implications for higher education. *Journal of Human Behavior in the Social Environment, 7*(1/2), 159-179.

Lehman, W., Greener, J., & Simpson, D. (2002). Assessing organizational readiness for change. *Journal of Substance Abuse Treatment, 22*(4), 197-210.

National Association of Social Workers. (1999). *Code of Ethics of the National Association of Social Workers*. Washington, DC: NASW Press.

Reid, W.J. (1987). Evaluating and intervention in developmental research. *Journal of Social Service Research, 11*(1), 17-36.

Roberts, A.R., & Yeager, K. (2004) *Evidence-Based Practice Manual: Research and Outcome Measures in Health and Human Services*. New York: Oxford University Press.

Rosen, A. (2003). Evidence-based social work practice: Challenges and promise. *Social Work Research, 27*(4), 197-208.

Rothman, J. (1992). Creating tools for intervention: The convergence of research methodologies. In A. Grasso & I. Epstein (Eds.), *Research Utilization in the Social Services*. New York: Haworth Press. 51-67.

Rothman, J. (1989). Intervention research: Application to runaway and homeless youth. *Social Work Research and Abstracts, 25*(1), 13-18.

Shackelford, K., Harper, M., Sullivan, K., & Edwards, T. (2005) Systematic case review data and child protective services outcomes: The development of the Mississippi model. *Journal of Evidence-Based Social Work* (this issue)

Simpson, D.D. (2002). A conceptual framework for transferring research to practice. *Journal of Substance Abuse Treatment, 22*(4), 171-182.

Southern Regional Quality Improvement Center (2001). *Summary of the Results of Needs Assessment*. University of Kentucky, College of Social Work.

Sundet, P., Mermelstein, J., & Watt, J.W. (2003). The role demonstration model of supervision. *Professional Development, 6*(2), 60-67.

Thomas, E.J. (1978). Generating innovation in social work: The paradigm of developmental research. *Journal of Social Service Research, 2*(1), 95-116.

Thyer, B. (2004). Science in evidence-based social work practice. In H. Briggs & T. Rzepnicki (Eds.). *Using Evidence in Social Work Practice*. Chicago, IL: Lyceum Books.

Thyer, B.A., & Wodarski, J.S. (Eds.). (1998). *Handbook of Empirical Social Work Practice*(Vol. I). New York: Wiley.

Usher, C.L., & Wildfire, J.B. (2003). Evidence-based practice in community-based child welfare systems. *Child Welfare, 82*(5), 597-614.

Webb, S. (2002). Evidence-based practice and decision analysis in social work: An implementation model. *Journal of Social Work, 2*(1), 45-63.

Wodarski, J.S., & Thyer, B.A. (Eds.). (1998). *Handbook of Empirical Social Work Practice*(Vol. II). New York: Wiley.

doi:10.1300/J394v04n03_11

Index

